And Suddenly, Everything Changed

Alan Twigg

This book is also available as an AudioBook

Editing by: Emmilysyoung

Copyright © 2019 Alan Twigg

All rights reserved.

CONTENTS

INTRODUCTION

<u>A word from the author:</u>

Until four years ago I was a normal middle-aged guy eating what I thought was a relatively healthy balanced diet. Basically, I was behaving more or less the same as everyone else that I knew.

But then my 18-year-old daughter intervened. She kept on nudging me and encouraging me to watch videos on Youtube, which I never did because, if I'm honest, I was worried that I would see and learn things that would force me into changes that I wasn't ready to make. Or so I believed.

And then it happened! It was the first day of a family holiday and I was just settling down next to the pool when my daughter slapped down a book next to me and said "Here you are Dad, I've bought this for you. I know health is important to you, so you need to read this."

I'm certainly not a bookworm, but I couldn't put it down. Within 5 days I had finished. And it was a big book! The undeniable and scientifically backed up facts and truths contained within conspired to change completely the way in which I saw the world and our society.

Since then I myself have been on a journey of discovery and a search of knowledge. It's really shocking you know, when you think you understand the world, when you believe that food holds no secrets and when you think that medicines and operations are the only way you can cure illnesses and diseases.

I wrote this audiobook to share my enthusiasm and passion with you and to encourage you and those you love, who may desperately need this knowledge, too, to consider change.

At the very least, this book will make you question your own assumptions and maybe add fuel to an already growing sense of curiosity about what is really going on.

It's a simple and entertaining story about a middle-aged guy who is about to experience the greatest paradigm shift of his life. His journey begins after a serious life-threating incident one day at work. In despair at what the future holds, Peter gradually awakens and discovers the shocking truth about something so commonplace we all believe it's normal, natural and necessary.

Along the way, Peter discovers that the path to health, peace and happiness is not where he thought it would be, so he follows a different, hidden path. On his journey we follow Peter as he meets the Nutritionist, the Marathon Runner, the Farmer, the Lads in the Pub, the Environmentalist and the Yogi. These intriguing and enlightened characters act as guides for Peter as they share their wisdom about lifestyle choices.

This book is for those looking to improve their health in a natural but incredibly powerful way. It's for those who have or know someone with heart disease, diabetes, lung disease, brain disease, digestive cancers, high-blood pressure, liver disease, kidney disease and almost any chronic illness.

But it's also a book for those who have already taken up a heart-healthy diet and lifestyle and discovered the core message of this book but are now looking to inspire or motivate a friend or loved one to make the change that they need.

Thank you. I hope it moves you.

CHAPTER 1 : PETER

"That it should come to this!" said Peter half laughing.

Peter always looked forward to making love to his wife, Susan. They'd been married for nearly 20 years, had raised two children together and he still found her incredibly attractive and appealing.

Tonight, right now, he wanted to feel her body, inhale her scent and experience a wonderful feeling of connection and contentment. Everything was perfect; they had just had a night out at their favourite restaurant and they were full of desire for each other. He was in the mood, and better still as far as Peter was concerned, so was she!

But it was not to be. His penis was limp, lifeless and - despite much encouragement from Susan - unmoving.

"I can't believe it," said Peter in frustration. He didn't feel like a real man. "I've only had the one pint of beer, bloody hell".

Little did Peter know that his inability to raise an erection was the first of a series of discoveries that would change his life completely. Bizarrely, he'd just received the greatest gift of his life. He just didn't know it yet.

The morning after the disappointing night before, Peter was in the kitchen drinking his usual morning coffee and making some lunch for later. His daughter Ellie, who was 13, was also up and about and getting ready for school.

"Dad," said Ellie, "What one change could we make today to help prevent climate change?"

"That's a tough one first thing in the morning," he replied. "I've only just opened my eyes and until I've drunk a cup of coffee, you're going to have to keep the questions very simple. Why do you want to know?"

"It's a project at school," said Ellie, "we have to come up with one change that we could do at home to help stop climate change. Oh yes, and it has to be cheap and easy to do."

"Well," Peter said, "it's your project so you're the one who needs to come up with something. Do you have any ideas?"

"Not really," said Ellie, but we don't have to hand it in yet"

"That gives you plenty of time then," said Dad.

It was only a 10-minute car journey from Peter's house to the sorting office where he started work every day at 8 am. He found himself thinking about the previous evening and his inability to… you know… get an erection. While it wasn't the first time he'd had trouble, it was the first time that it had failed completely despite being in the mood. *Maybe I'm impotent*, he thought to himself. Peter knew that some of his mates had already started taking Viagra. It was a popular subject once the beer got flowing when he met up with his mates once a month. Some of his friends even seemed quite proud of themselves that they could buy a pill that gave them super-human erections. He'd always thought that it was a sad state of affairs that they needed to be taking medication in to get a hard on.

Until today, Peter hadn't been ready to accept that he couldn't get an erection anymore and that perhaps it was time for him to join his mates and turn to the Viagra. As he drove into the car park, he thought about bringing up his erection troubles with his mates in the in the pub after a few beers the next time he was out with the lads. He laughed to himself as he contemplated the 'friendly' advice he could expect from his mates after they'd all drunk a few beers.

Peter worked at the post office. He used to deliver the post by foot, but he now preferred to drive around in a van and simply pick up the mail and take it to the sorting office. For him the job was like the film "Groundhog Day". Easy, secure, and undemanding. Each day was the same as the next. The pay was unremarkable, but in return he experienced no stress, the work was incredibly straightforward, and his daily work routine was unchanging.

He'd park up, get out of the car and walk through the main doors into the warehouse before crossing the huge floor area to reach the drink's machine, which was located at the other end. He'd get a coffee from the machine and pass the time of day with whoever happened to be there. From the drink's machine, he'd walk over to the dispatch counter to collect the keys for one of the post vans. He'd usually get the same van and the same route. His job was simply to drive to the various pillar boxes, post offices and local business to collect the post that needed bringing back to the sorting office.

In fact, his job was so routine and simple that he'd often get so lost in his thoughts that he'd sometimes get back to the sorting office before realizing that he'd actually forgotten to empty a pillar box or two or forgotten to pick up some sacks from one of the businesses.

Today had started in the same way as always.

One of his colleagues - known to everyone as "Double Chips" - was standing at the drink's machine. Peter didn't know Double Chips' real name; all he knew was that he'd got his unflattering nickname after always ordering double of everything from the fast-food takeaways. When Peter had first started at the post office, "Double Chips" had actually been slim and fit. That was in the days when the both of them had delivered the post by foot and carried a heavy bag around with them for miles and miles every day in Sheffield, one England's hilliest cities. But ever since switching to the van, "Double Chips" had put on lots of weight and his neck had all but disappeared into his body. Peter had also become a lot heavier and was certainly a lot less fit, but compared to Double Chips, he considered his overall health and fitness to be OK for a man in his 50s.

After collecting the keys for the van, Peter drove out of the sorting office gate and as usual made a beeline to his favourite café for breakfast. It was located on the corner of a busy junction and was just your typical friendly café.

"Morning, Peter. The usual?" "Yes, please, Cath. I'll be in my spot!". A few minutes later Cath arrived at his table with his usual of bacon, scrambled eggs, mushrooms, beans and a couple of slices of toast together with another cup of coffee. "How's the family" said Cath setting his breakfast down on the table in front of him. "Fine", said Peter. Ellie's got this homework project about climate change. But you look out of the window and all the parents are carting their kids to school in great, big SUVs. The world's gone mad! Why does everyone want to drive around in a tank anyway?" None of that nonsense when we were kids," Cath replied. "We walked to school every day. Kept us busy as well as healthy." "You're right there", Peter said.

Peter left the café, got back in the van, and set off for his first port of call, picking up sacks of post and parcels from an engineering company near the town centre.

"Morning," said Peter, entering the main entrance.

"Morning" said the friendly receptionist. "There are two sacks for you on the second floor, but you'll have to use the stairs because the lift is broken and we're waiting for it to get repaired".

Bloody hell, thought Peter to himself, *those sacks will be heavy*. Fifteen kilograms was the maximum allowed weight of each sack. But he knew from experience that they were likely to be much heavier.

Peter needed to put in much more effort than usual to climb the flights of stairs to the second floor. His breath was short and he was struggling. He was startled. Never before had he been out of breath like this. Peter took a short break at the top of the first flight before continuing to climb the second. Each step was heavy, almost as though he was carrying a heavy load, but he was empty handed. He didn't feel well.

Waiting at the top of the stairs were the two sacks of post. Just as Peter had expected, they both easily weighed more than the 15 kilograms allowed. It was a busy building, but there was no one else around. He asked himself whether he should try to carry both sacks at once, or one at a time? As he lifted the first, his mind was made up for him. It was heavy! Only the one for now, then.

Just as on the way up, the way down the stairs and out to his van parked in front of the building required much more effort than usual. He was struggling to catch his breath and slightly dizzy. For a moment, he considered whether he should tell the receptionist that he couldn't climb the stairs again to collect the second sack. Should he call in sick at the sorting office?

His pride, however, got the better of him. He set off again to collect the remaining sack from the second floor. Climbing the stairs again was even more difficult than it had been the first-time round. On reaching the sack he took a break to recover and with all his effort and willpower engaged somehow managed to bring the second sack down, but the situation was about to worsen.

As Peter heaved the sack into the back of the van, he suddenly felt nauseated and dizzy. All he wanted was to lie down. There was room in the back with the post bags, so - with the swing doors open - he just laid himself down. He was sweating. He could take shallow breaths in, but he couldn't fill his lungs.

Peter was frightened.

"Are you alright?" said the receptionist, who had come out to where Peter was. "I think so", said Peter, lying. "Those sacks were bloody heavy. I'll be right enough in a few minutes". "Are you sure", she said. Peter nodded. "We'll I'm just inside if you need me", she said.

What should he do now?, he thought to himself. Should he call in at work and tell them what had happened? Should he go straight to the doctors? He closed his eyes and concentrated on his breathing, trying to bring it back to a normal rhythm. He was conscious that the receptionist was watching him so after a few minutes he raised his head and sat up in the back of the van.

Through the glass façade of the building he could see that the receptionist was wearing a concerned face. He pulled his mobile from his pocket and called in at work, telling the dispatch office that he wasn't feeling well. He'd come back to the sorting office with the van and then go home. He still felt lightheaded as he got into the driver's seat. Luckily, he'd not come far and it was only a few minutes back to the depot. In all the years he'd worked at the post office, he'd never gone home early and had been seldom off work due to illness.

Driving home after dropping off the post van and now feeling a little better, he wondered what he would tell Susan. He opened the door and noticed that the washing up needed doing, but he was suddenly hit by a feeling of weakness again. He just didn't have the strength to do anything more strenuous than lying on the sofa.

"What are you doing home?" said Susan, as she came through the door after returning home from work. Until now, Peter had told no one about his fright this morning. But he'd made up his mind to tell his wife. He knew what she would say.

"You'll have to go and get checked out," she said. "Urgently".

CHAPTER 2 : THE CARDIOLOGIST

Peter's doctor referred him straight to the cardiologist. On his second visit, he was due to have a coronary angiography.

"Dr Newton's getting the room ready, Said the nurse, "but we just need to check over your forms. How have you been feeling since your last appointment?"

"Alright," Peter said. It was mostly true; he'd been thinking a lot about the incident he'd had at work and if, perhaps, he had some kind of heart disease, and what that would mean for him. He had a family, a job, a life! He was only 53 years old, for god's sake! Sure, he was a little overweight and didn't exercise as much as he should, but he didn't smoke, only drank at weekends and ate what he considered to be a balanced diet.

"Yeah," he said. "It's been alright."

The nurse lifted her clipboard.

"You mentioned last time that your grandfather died after suffering a heart attack?"

"Yes, he was 73."

"And your father as well?"

"He was diagnosed with heart disease at the age of... 63, I think. He had stents, then a by heart bypass surgery a couple of years later. Perhaps heart disease just runs in the family and there's nothing we can do about it."

"Let's wait and see what Dr Newton says, shall we? We gleaned a lot from your ECG and your stress test last time. Now have you eaten in the past 4 hours this morning?"

"No, I had a light breakfast about 5.30."

"You had a shower?"

"Yes."

"Good, that lowers the risk of infection."

He knew. He'd read and re-read that leaflet over and over since his last appointment.

"Have you drunk anything but water this morning?" the nurse continued.

"Only water for me."

"Excellent. A model patient. Dr Newton will call you in shortly."

"Everything's ready for you," said Dr. Newton. "If you'd like to come through, we can begin."

It had been explained to Peter that the procedure would take around 30 minutes and involved a long thin flexible tube being threaded up into the heart and coronary arteries where a dye would be released. Using X-ray images, any narrowing of the coronary arteries would show up and a diagnosis could be made.

Peter hoped that it was something and nothing and that he would be able to return to his normal life soon. After the procedure, Peter was told to relax, rest, and drink plenty of water and await Dr. Newton with the results. It wasn't long before he reappeared with a file in his hand.

"How are you feeling?" asked Dr. Newton, taking a chair next to Peter as he lay resting from the procedure.

"Nervous," Peter replied. He didn't like the doctor's poker face.

"It's bad news I'm afraid," said Dr. Newton. "You have two blockages and one narrowing of the coronary arteries. I don't think I need to emphasise how serious this could be. I recommend heart bypass surgery to restore blood supply to your heart muscle."

Although Peter knew that this was a possibility, he was still shocked to hear the diagnosis. He felt a sense of loss as though Dr. Newton had just taken something away from him that he had taken for granted for so long. His health. It dawned on Peter that he didn't like the thought of not being fully healthy and able. What would Susan and Ellie think? Would they think him less of a husband and father because of his illness?

"Do you have any questions?" asked Dr. Newton.

"Is a heart operation really necessary? What will happen if I don't go for surgery?" Peter asked.

"If the blood supply to the heart muscle continues to decrease as a result of increasing obstruction of a coronary artery, you may have a myocardial infarction or heart attack. If the blood flow cannot be restored to the particular area of the heart muscle affected, the tissue dies. You need surgery", said Dr. Newton.

"When?" enquired Peter.

"Your operation will most likely take place within the next six months, maybe less if you are lucky. Until then I'm going to prescribe Aspirin and ask you to take it easy. Don't exert yourself too much and try to keep your breathing regular. Don't overdo it". Said Dr. Newton.

Peter thanked the doctor as he left, his mind still reeling from the news. How was he going to break this news to Susan? He'd have to rip off the band-aid.

"You need a triple heart bypass!," said Susan, "I can't believe it - you're only in your fifties!"

"Neither can I," said Peter. "I really don't fancy the thought of having my chest sawn open. Do you realise they'll take veins out of my legs and stitch them onto my heart, like some crazy plumbing job? I wish there was another way, but the Doctor said it was this or a heart attack."

Strangely, Peter felt a sense of embarrassment by having to tell Susan the news. He'd always regarded himself as strong and healthy and this revelation had changed his own perception of himself. Had it changed Susan's perception of him?

"Do you think I've got this because of something I've done or not done or just in my genes like my Dad and his Dad", said Peter. To be honest", said Susan, "I'm not sure. You've put on quite a bit of weight since you stopped walking at work. You used to play golf and squash regularly, too, but now you hardly go at all."

"I suppose so" Peter replied, "I must admit that I feel more stressed than before and I've been getting upset about stupid things. And we've both noticed that I can't manage a hard on anymore. So are you saying you think it's a lack of exercise that's brought this on?". "I've no idea, said Susan, it's just that I've noticed a change in you since you got the van at work, so it might be connected, who knows?"

"I'm sure you'll be alright after the operation", said Susan. "Maybe you can come to the yoga classes with me afterwards, I love it and I think it would be good for us both to do something together, don't you think?"

"You really enjoy going there don't you, said Peter, are there any other men there apart from the instructor?"

"There's a guy called Michael who never misses", said Susan, "I think it would be perfect for you as well, It's not just about stretching you know. We always start with breathing exercises and meditation and I know it's help me to feel more relaxed and at ease. I know you've always told me to get lost in the past when I've asked you to come along, but maybe you could reconsider after you've recovered."

Peter was just thinking it over when Susan suddenly raised her voice and said "Michael. "Michael in our yoga class runs marathons now."

"So?" said Peter.

"He told me that he'd been diagnosed with heart disease three years ago and had been told he needed surgery, too, but never had it."

"What and he's running marathons now?" said Peter. "How did he manage that?

"I don't know," said Susan. "Maybe you should meet him and find out. He'll be there on Friday."

CHAPTER 3 : THE MARATHON RUNNER

Have I really agreed to go with Susan to Yoga? he asked himself. What if someone sees? I'll have to tell them it's only to meet this Michael bloke. The plan was to wait until after the class had finished to speak to him. The words 'clutching at straws' had sprung to Peter's mind. On the other hand, meeting up with Michael and hearing his story couldn't make matters worse; after all, from what Susan had said it sounded like Michael had been in a similar situation to him three years ago. He supposed it wouldn't hurt to hear him out.

She'd suggested that Peter might as well take part while he was there, but he'd refused, as usual.

Instead Peter went for a walk and arrived back at the yoga hall around 10 minutes before the class was due to finish. The yoga hall was a wooden building with a sloped tiled roof and a mainly glass frontage. From outside where Peter was standing, it was easy to see what was going on inside. There were approximately 12 taking part in the yoga class this evening and they were all sitting cross legged with their backs to Peter. Apart from the instructor there was only one other man. As the yoga lesson ended the participants made their way out and Susan introduced him. "Hi," said Michael smiling and reaching out his hand. "Susan tells me that you'd like to have a chat about my miraculous recovery from heart disease."

"Yes, that's right," said Peter. "Susan said that you didn't have surgery and that you're now running marathons. I've just been told that I've got heart disease and that I need a triple heart bypass. So I thought it would be nice to talk to you and find out how you managed it. To be honest, I've just been watching you through the window and you certainly don't paint a picture of someone who'd get heart disease."

"Shall we talk while we make our way to the car park", said Susan, it's a good 10-minute walk." "OK", said Michael.

"Three years ago, I didn't look or feel like I do now," said Michael. "I've transformed into a far better version of myself since my heart scare. It all started in January. I'd just made a New Year's resolution to get myself fit. I'd always wanted to run a marathon, but I'd become overweight, had no energy and was sick of the way I looked and felt. I was out on my very first training run when I suddenly got a crushing pain in the chest. It was horrible. I went to the doctor and he told me that I had heart disease and I'd need a bypass."

"But you never had one?" said Peter, who was starting to feel short of breath again. "Can we walk a bit slower, I'm struggling a bit".

"Of course," said Michael. "No, I never had the OP. There was no way I was just going to go under the knife, pop some pills, and basically give up on my dream of running a marathon. I was determined to find another way. There had to be an alternative. It was while leaving the hospital that I was handed a leaflet. The front said, 'Are you getting healthy or just treating the symptoms? Speak to the Nutritionist.' Like I said, I was on a mission to find another way, so I called the number and made an appointment with Gail. What she told me changed my life."

"What did she tell you?" said Peter, a little too quickly.

"Where do I start? She's incredible. She's got this whole new way of looking at food and diet that I'd never experienced before. Also her own story of how she became a nutritionist is really interesting. Everything changed for me after that. I've got her number, maybe you can see her yourself?", said Michael.

"Sure, I'd like that," Peter said. "So what happened to you after that?"

"After speaking to the nutritionist," said Michael, "I felt a huge surge of motivation. She'd given me a plan and a new paradigm. But I still had heart disease, I was still on Aspirin, and I was still scheduled for a heart bypass. I decided to continue with my goal of running a marathon. I wanted to have a goal. I would just have to start training at a far slower pace. I put on my running shoes and began to *walk*. My goal was to walk a mile each day at the beginning and to increase very slowly the distance and speed each week. At the same time, I incorporated all of the things that Gail had told me into my daily life and waited to see whether I would notice any improvements."

"And did you?" asked Peter.

"Each day I seemed able to go a little further and a little faster," said Michael. "After just a month I was managing to break into a couple of minutes of slow jogging. And my breathing seemed to be improving, too. I was still scheduled for a heart bypass, so I went back to see the Cardiologist and he confirmed that my blood tests, stress tests and overall heart health were improving. I decided to push on. And I kept on improving. After three months, continuous improvement, commitment and belief, I decided to delay my planned heart operation.

"I'd be worried about doing that", said Peter. "It sounds a bit risky to me." By now the three of them had reached the car park and were standing next to Peter and Susan's car. "To be honest", said Susan, it also sounds a bit risky to me, too, I'd be unhappy if Peter decided to put off his operation."

"You're both right, normally I wouldn't have done it either. But I'd come a long way and felt that I was making real progress. It was at about this time that I learnt about the role that stress plays in heart disease," said Michael. "That's when I started yoga, which you'll find out if you go and visit Gail, fitted perfectly with the changes that I'd already made. Yoga made me realize just how inflexible I'd become over the years. Sitting cross-legged for even 5-minutes was very uncomfortable at first. Yet for all the discomfort, it was the benefits that were more striking. Yoga was making me feel calmer and slowing me down. I was in less of a rush. The breathing and stretching exercises helped my running as well. I could run faster and longer without getting out of breath.

"After 18 months, I was ready to enter my first half-marathon. I've now run two full marathons and I'm even beginning to consider training for my first half-Iron Man."

"That's… incredible. Honestly, it's really inspiring," said Peter.

"I can give you the contact details of Gail, the nutritionist, if you want," said Michael. "But don't get your hopes up too much."

"Why?" said Peter. After all that, he could feel his hopes already rising.

"It's one thing to have the information," said Michael, "but it's another thing to put that knowledge into practice. I had a goal. I wanted to run. This was the thing that motivated me to make the changes that led to my improvement. Without a goal, I'm not sure that I would be where I am today. Do you have a goal?"

"To get better," said Peter.

"I'm sorry", said Michael. "But I don't think that will be enough."

Susan felt a drop of rain hit her hand. Looking up to the sky she said "It's starting to rain, I think we'd better get off".

"Thank you for sharing your story with us" said Peter. "It's given me something to think about and a little bit of hope."

"You're welcome", said Michael. "I hope it works out for you. See you next time Susan".

Driving home with Susan, Peter started to wonder what Michael had meant about him needing a goal. He thought about his goals and it was then that he realized that, apart from getting better, he didn't have any. Perhaps this trip had been in vain after all. He supposed there was no harm in seeing the nutritionist anyway and taking it from there.

CHAPTER 4 : THE NUTRITIONIST

"Nice to meet you, I'm Peter."

"Hello, I'm Gail."

Gail stretched out a soft hand to Peter as he took a seat. Her consulting room was different from anything Peter had seen before. The furniture and decorations were eastern and there were lots of plants the whole space seemed to be in constant contact with nature. Wood had also been used for the flooring and windows. An inviting scent hung in the air, but Peter couldn't quite place it. Was it lavender? Maybe chamomile? He'd not expected anything like this and yet it was comforting.

"To be honest, I don't really know what I'm doing here," said Peter. "I've always eaten a very balanced diet."

Gail paused, looked at Peter in the eye, and waited a second or two before questioning him.

"Really? I understand that you have been diagnosed with heart disease and that the recommendation is for a triple bypass operation, is that correct?"

"That's right," said Peter.

"And why do you think you got heart disease?" asked Gail.

"Just bad luck, I suppose," said Peter. "My Dad and his dad both had heart disease so I guess it's just in my genes."

"When talking about the main drivers and risk factors for heart disease - and, indeed, many other modern chronic diseases - diet and lifestyle are far more important than genes. What do you hope to get out of our appointment today?"

Peter squirmed in his seat.

"I don't want surgery," said Peter. "I met Michael the other day, a patient of yours. He told me that you helped him avoid surgery. Did you know he's running marathons now? He recommended I come and see you, too."

"Are you prepared to make significant dietary and lifestyle changes in order to avoid surgery and to return to health?"

"Yes," said Peter, confidently. Then he thought back to Michael's words, about having a goal in mind and that perhaps he didn't have one. Gail seemed sceptical of him, too. He looked her in the eyes. "You don't seem convinced."

"Lots of people come to see me, Peter," said Gail, "many of them in worse health than you. Most tell me that they are ready and willing to make changes in their lives. But only a small minority actually follow through."

"Like Michael," said Peter.

"Exactly," Gail said. "Most people are looking for a simple and easy solution that doesn't involve real change. Many people would rather risk their lives and have major heart surgery than change their diet and introduce a little physical exercise into their lives. Habit change - especially in regard to food - is a tough ask for many. It's such a shame, because the diet I recommend does not involve going hungry at all. In fact, you can eat as much as you want, provided you're eating the foods that I recommend. There are so many delicious foods that you can eat that it's far more likely that your choice will expand rather than decrease."

"Michael told me you have a story of your own about how you came to be a nutritionist," said Peter, inviting a reply.

"Well, for many years I was a GP," said Gail. "I entered the medical profession because I wanted to help people get well. But over time I began to think more and more that while I was helping people manage their diseases, I wasn't helping them to recover their health, which is what I wanted. I would prescribe pills and refer patients to specialists and their symptoms would improve, but I didn't feel as though I was getting to the root causes.

"Then one day, one of my patients who'd been diagnosed with type 2 diabetes told me that he'd heard that his disease could be cured with diet alone. I told him that as far as I knew this wasn't possible. Then he asked me something that made me question my own professional knowledge. *How much education did you receive about the way diet and lifestyle affect health*? I had to admit that I had virtually none. I'd never really thought about it.

"When I got home, I started to do some digging and straightaway found an article reporting that medical students claimed that they learned nothing about nutrition. Nothing! They said what they are taught is not practical or relevant to most of the medical problems they see in GP surgeries, clinics and hospitals. This was something to which I could relate. That article led me to more research and I found Dr Michael Mosely, who talked about nutrition not being a part of traditional medical school training. He never learnt it a decade or two ago, and now his son currently at medical school isn't learning about it either. I looked into it myself. It's the same all over the USA, all over Europe. That's nothing short of unbelievable!"

"I always thought doctors knew all about food and what you need to eat", said Peter.

"As strange as it seems, so did I" said Gail. "I wanted to find out more so I kept on reading and researching and, if I'm honest, got a little obsessed with finding out more. It turns out that even the most conservative and traditional of health authorities all agree that diet is an important risk factor for the development of most of our most common modern diseases including heart disease, strokes and type 2 diabetes. Others sources say that diet and lifestyle account for up to 90% of all heart disease cases."

"90 percent", said Peter with surprise in his voice, repeating Gail's words. "So it could be the way I've been living that's caused my heart disease?"

"Most probably, yes", said Gail. It's unbelievable isn't it that I and most of the medical community receive no formal training or education on nutrition.

So I carried on and the more I searched, the more I uncovered research paper after research paper supporting the seeming ability of diet to prevent - and in many cases also to treat - many of our leading killers."

Gail paused and walked over to her desk. She opened the drawer and pulled out a thin bundle of papers before taking a few steps over to Peter and handing them to him. Peter took the papers from Gail and looked down. On the front it said in big letters *THE LANCET*. Underneath there was a title, which read *"Can lifestyle changes reverse coronary heart disease?* Underneath that it read *Reprinted from the Lancet, Saturday 21ˢᵗ July 1990.*

"What's this?", asked Peter.

"In my opinion this is one of the most ground-breaking and most unheard-of set of findings ever published in the field of nutrition. The author is Dean Ornish and he carried out a randomized trial that showed that patients with heart disease that were treated with diet and lifestyle changes improved. There was also a control group, whose conditions got worse and worse. This was the first time that diet and lifestyle changes alone had been proven to not only stop, but also to reverse heart disease."

"So you're saying that this article shows that food can cure heart disease?", said Peter.

"With some other lifestyle changes, yes", said Gail. "And that's not all. I've discovered that diet and lifestyle alone can also help to prevent and, in many cases, reverse the top killers of our age including, cancer, stroke, lung disease, Alzheimer's disease, digestive disorders, kidney disorders and diabetes?" Gail said, counting them off on her fingers.

"Eventually, I became so convinced of the benefits of nutrition, diet and lifestyle changes on health that I decided to become a nutritionist. Like I said, I felt so out of balance as a GP that I was ready to embrace a big change of direction in my career anyway. For the last five years I've been helping people to regain their health. Michael is a shining example."

It was a lot to take in, but Peter something akin to resolve.

"How can you help me?" asked Peter.

"Well, first you have to commit to making significant changes in your diet and lifestyle," said Gail. "For one, it means that you'll need to embrace a purely plant-based diet. Instead of meat, fish, bacon, milk, cheese, and eggs, you'll be eating beans, wholegrains, and lots of vegetables and fruit."

"For how long?" asked Peter.

"If you don't want your heart disease to get worse and you want to give yourself the best chance of a healthy life - *forever*," said Gail.

"That sounds a bit extreme", said Peter.

Gail paused.

"Many would consider having your chest opened with a saw and having veins removed from your leg so they can be stitched onto your heart as extreme," replied Gail, "but I do understand your point of view. That's why I asked you earlier if you were prepared to make significant changes. As I explained earlier, many are just not prepared to make the changes necessary. For them, the prospect of surgery and drugs for the rest of their lives is preferable to the prospect of not eating their favourite foods, which, by the way, are often the very foods that helped create the disease in the first place.

"I can tell you a few things that might help you," said Gail. "Firstly, almost all the people that I see that go onto make successful changes in their lives are the ones with a larger goal. They know why they want to get better. Take Michael, for instance; his goal was to run a marathon. So when I told him that there might be chance to return to health without surgery and drugs, he grabbed the opportunity with both hands. Secondly, like most others, now your focus is on the foods that you'll not be able to eat rather than on all the new and delicious foods that you'll discover. And, thirdly, if you decide to follow my advice and the diet and lifestyle recommendations that I give you, you'll discover harmony in your life."

Now she's sounding like a hippy, thought Peter. But then he remembered just how fit Michael had looked and how sure he'd been. Who was he to judge? He was here because he had heart disease, after all.

"I have some questions," said Peter.

"Fire away."

"If what you are saying is true, why didn't the cardiologist mention diet or lifestyle to me?"

"Remember," said Gail, "that nutrition and lifestyle interventions are not taught in medical school. The cardiologist most probably simply doesn't know. And even if he does know about nutrition and diet, many practitioners simply don't believe that patients will implement dietary changes into their lives. Doctors have busy schedules and full surgeries. Why spend considerable time explaining diet and exercise to their patients when the patient is unlikely to follow the advice anyway? Sadly, I must confess that I witnessed this all too often in my own patients. Nevertheless, I strongly believe that if an alternative exists, the patient should be told about it and allowed to make up their own mind."

"I have another question" said Peter. "No meat or fish. Where will I get my protein?"

"Great question," said Gail. "It's very easy for a plant-based diet to meet the recommendations for protein. Nearly all vegetables, beans, grains, nuts, and seeds contain protein. People eating varied diets containing vegetables, beans, grains, nuts, and seeds have no difficulty getting enough protein. So you don't need to worry about that. It's a myth. Can I ask *you* a question? Where do you get your fibre?"

Peter looked puzzled.

"If you're an average person, your diet only contains 60% of the recommended official daily amount," said Gail. "If you decide to follow my advice, you'll be consuming far more fibre, which is associated with reduced cholesterol levels, reduced blood sugar, increased mineral absorption, weight management, reduced inflammation and much more. There are so many benefits associated with a strictly plant-based diet, it's impossible to go through them all with you now. But I can recommend a book for you to read and a film that you can watch for free on YouTube if you're interested."

"Alright, could you write them down for me?" said Peter.

"Of course," said Gail, taking a sticky note from her pad and writing as she spoke. "The book is called *How Not to Die* by Dr. Michael Greger – I know it sounds a little dramatic, but it's fantastic. The film is called *What the Health*. Here you are."

Peter took the note and thanked her. Perhaps the title *was* a little dramatic, but he himself was facing the prospect of heart surgery or death, so it wouldn't hurt to take a look. Any other options were welcome.

"You'll also need to exercise," said Gail. "Have you ever been a sporty type?"

"I used to play squash and golf. In fact, I used to walk everyday delivering the post before I switched to the van around five years ago. I don't play squash anymore and I only go golfing now and again because the group I play with want to go round the course driving a golf cart rather than walking. For me, playing golf in a buggy is not really golf."

"That sounds encouraging", said Gail, "You have a hobby that could involve physical activity if you walked and carried your clubs and you have a job that you could perhaps also leverage to be more active. To get physically healthy, you don't need to enter into an extreme training regime like Michael did; people can often get all the activity that they need just by making simple changes. In your case, I'd recommend that you start with walking. Just go for a walk once a day and each time you do, see if you can increase the distance and the intensity by just a little. Time is a fascinating thing. One of my favourite Zen sayings is, *in nature nothing is hurried, yet everything is achieved.*

"Most people rush out and try to do things too quickly. Our society has conditioned us to want instant gratification. This even extends into the realms of exercise and learning. I remember when I wanted to learn German and went looking for a book", laughed Gail. "I remember books with titles like *"Learn to Speak German Quickly in Just 7 Days"*.

"But that is not the way of nature. In nature, progress is usually slow, but leads to abundance and completeness. I want you to embrace this in your life, Peter. Start slow. Even increasing your walk by just one minute per week can make a difference. Even if you started walking for just a minute a day and increased it by another minute each week, by the end of the year you'd be walking for 52 minutes. You can apply this gentle but powerful approach to anything. It's beautiful, enabling your body, your heart and mind to adapt slowly and gradually. Adding a minute each week is easy. On the other hand, going for a 52-minute run right off the bat would be gruelling. Patience and being in harmony with nature is the key."

Peter didn't know what to make of this new information. Of course, he'd expected to be told that he'd need to make some dietary changes, but he wasn't sure that he was ready to base his entire diet around plants. It sounded very drastic.

"I can see that you have doubts," said Gail. "My advice to you would be to take the time to think over what we have discussed this afternoon. I think the most important first step is to work out why you want to be healthy and to develop a clear long-term goal for your life. Having a clear objective and purpose will give you the energy and motivation you need to make the little but important healthy choices daily."

Leaving the nutritionist's office, Peter felt as though he was being pointed away from what he knew and accepted. Could it really be that his health could improve by eating a plant-based diet and exercising more? *It all sounds too good to be true*, Peter thought to himself. But his thoughts kept returning to the image of Michael and the nagging feeling that he was still missing something. Apparently, if he was to make this work, he would need a goal as well. *Maybe it would be easier to just have the bypass operation and take the pills?* he thought as he drove home.

He'd barely passed the threshold when he was waylaid by his youngest.

"Dad," said Ellie, "can we go and buy two new shower heads?"

"What? Why?" said Peter, closing the front door behind him.

"There's one I found that uses less water and less heating, which is good for the environment," said Ellie.

"I suppose so," said Peter, wearily, "but I've a lot on my plate right now, so you'll have to wait a couple of days."

Peter found Susan waiting in the living room. She turned down the TV and listened as Peter told her of Gail and the proposed changes.

"What do you think?" said Peter.

"Well," said Susan, "it's up to you. A vegetarian diet is part of yoga, so I suppose we could go a step further and try to cut out dairy as well. Do you genuinely want to give it a try?"

"I'm not sure," said Peter. "She was a bit too *woo-woo* at times for me."

"I've got an idea," said Susan. "Let's go down to the pub for a meal and a drink and see if they've got anything on the menu that fits the bill, what do you think? You don't have to decide right now."

"Good idea, I could murder a drink," said Peter.

"Shall we walk it to the Sportsman so that we can start your exercise regime at the same time", said Susan with a giggle.

"Good idea", said Peter. He knew there was a slim chance that one or two his friends might be there having a drink. *I hope I don't bump into any of them*, he thought to himself, *I'm not in the mood for jokes at my expense tonight.*

It was a quiet night in the Sportsman and Susan and Peter sat down at an empty table and both took a menu from the holder in the middle.

"There's nothing on here that I fancy, apart from the steak," said Peter.

"They have a lasagne and a five-bean chili that both tick all of the boxes," said Susan.

"OK," said Peter, reluctantly, "I'll try the chili."

Looking through the various options on the menu, Peter was noticing for the first time that virtually all the options contained either meat, fish, or dairy. *This is going to be really tough*, thought Peter to himself.

Susan, however, saw this as an opportunity for her and Peter to pull together and as a chance for Peter to get well again without having to undergo surgery. But she also knew Peter well enough to know that he was a creature of habit and that he'd need her support if he was going to pull it off.

"What do you think to cooking something veggie tomorrow?" said Susan.

"Not a lot", said Peter.

"It sounds like you've given up already and you've not even made it past one evening meal," said Susan. "There are thousands of recipes online, you could pick one and cook it."

"I hate cooking," said Peter.

Susan thought it was important that Peter got involved so she said, "I'll do you a deal. You go and get the ingredients from High Valley Farm tomorrow and I'll cook it, what do you say?"

"High Valley is a dairy farm," said Peter.

"Not anymore," said Susan.

CHAPTER 5 : THE FARMER

"Right then," said Susan, checking her list. "I'll be needing lentils, carrots, sweet potatoes, onion, garlic, mushrooms, celery and tomatoes. You should be able to get them all from the farm shop.

"What's it going to be?" asked Peter, sceptical.

"It's going to be a lentil stew," said Susan, "I'm making a big pot of it so we can have it the day after, too, and maybe freeze some for another day."

High Valley Farm was only five minutes' drive away. Peter had known it since he was a kid; it had been one of his favourite spots for sledging in the winter snow, as it was located at the bottom of a very steep hill. The fields that surrounded the farmhouse had always been grazed by cows, but as he drew near today, he couldn't make out any cattle at all. Instead, he could see that two large greenhouses had been constructed. It looked like some of the fields were even being allowed to return to their natural state.

As he pulled into the newly-constructed entrance, there was a large sign with the words, *Welcome to High Valley Farm – Kind Organic Food and Café*. The driveway and the parking spaces had been recently improved and he could see that the farmhouse had been extended to accommodate the shop and café. *They've done a good job of this*, thought Peter to himself. The farm shop was built out of timber and had a protruding terrace supported by wooden pillars. The terrace was being used to keep the rain and worst of the weather off the entrance area.

Just as much effort had been put into the inside of the shop. All the fruits and veggies were displayed in wicker baskets. Wow, thought Peter to himself, it all looks delicious. Every shade and colour seemed to be represented and there was a wonderfully fresh scent as well. It was a nice place to be.

The words "Farm News" adorned a large blackboard. Empty spaces on the walls had been decorated either with images of lush fruit and vegetables or what Peter considered to be provocative messages such as, *You know you are not an animal lover when their body parts are in your shopping trolley* or *Animals are Not Ingredients*.

"Morning," said a friendly voice. "Welcome to our shop."

"Morning!" said Peter, turning to greet the smiling man at the counter. He pointed to one of the signs he'd just read on the wall. "That's a bit extreme, isn't it?"

"Not to me," said the man laughing. "I was the one who put it there. My name's David, my family and I are the owners of the farm and shop. You are?"

"Nice to meet you, David. I'm Peter."

"Is this your first time here?" he asked.

"Yes, is it that obvious?" said Peter, chuckling. "The missus is cooking and I'm here to get the ingredients."

"You know, only ten years ago, I would have found those signs provocative and completely out of order, too," said David. "But I realize now how misguided I was and today I'm trying to make up for the harm and pain that I caused."

"What do you mean?" said Peter.

"Do you really want to know?", asked David.

Peter was a little surprised by this question and, if truth be known, a little reluctant. Yesterday, he'd listened to the nutritionist as she'd told him lots of things about food that he hadn't heard before; now he had the sense that the farmer was about to tell him things that he might not want to hear as well. Should he decline or should he listen?

"To be honest, I'm not really sure", said Peter, "but something tells me I should say yes".

"I promise it's a great story, Peter," David said, resting on the counter top. "My journey started just over ten years ago when I inherited the dairy farm from my parents. Growing up on the farm, I'd learned all about how a farm works. When I left school, it was clear that I would just continue working in the family business. It was expected of me and to be honest I'd never really questioned it or thought about an alternative career. So ten years ago, the farm became mine. Now it was entirely up to me to run it and ultimately to take the decisions about its future. I don't know… there was something about being responsible for the farm, the animals and the future of both that triggered a change in me. At first the feeling was very subtle, like a nagging doubt. I started very gradually to question some of the things that we were doing on the farm. I'd not voiced any of my doubts to my family - I have a wife and two young daughters - but week by week and month by month my questions and the uncomfortable feeling in my conscience began to grow."

David stopped speaking and raised his eyes to meet Peter's. "I think cows have emotions," he said. "They can sense when they are going to be killed. You can tell if they are happy, sad, bored, and you can tell there's something going on behind the eyes. Cows, like all animals, are sentient beings."

The way in which David spoke had got Peter hooked into the story, but he had his doubts about that last statement. "I think the idea of cows having emotions is a bit silly", said Peter.

David paused for a moment before continuing with his story.

"When a dairy cow is no longer productive after around three years, she is sent for slaughter and the meat used for beef. That means that trucks arrive at the farm to collect them and to take them to the slaughterhouse. I began to dread the day the animal transporters would arrive. And after they had gone, I began to feel a sense of shame and betrayal. Unfortunately, for me that was only the tip of the iceberg, because I had also started to question the morality of milk and cheese. Most people are unaware of what it takes to produce milk and from it cheese. Many people think that cows just graze in the field and produce milk, but the truth is very different and hidden from the public in a very systematic way, otherwise I'm sure more people would question the morality of it all."

"But cows do graze in fields and then give milk, don't they?" said Peter.

"Yes, some cows do graze in fields and yes, all cows are kept for their milk production," replied David. "But getting a continuous supply of milk from the cow can only be achieved through what amounts to systemic cruelty. This part is… shocking. Most people don't like to hear it. Are you sure you want me to go on?"

Peter nodded, captured in the story.

"A mother cow only produces milk when she gets pregnant. So, starting from the age of fifteen months, she will usually be artificially inseminated. Farmers mechanically draw semen from a bull, and then force the female cow into a narrow trap, known as a "cattle crush", where they will forcefully impregnate her. When she gives birth, her calf will typically be removed within 36 hours, so the farmers can steal and sell you the milk that is meant for her baby. Wildlife experts say that a strong bond between cow and calf is formed quickly after birth. Following that callous separation, the mother will bellow and scream for days, wondering where her baby is. The answer depends on the gender of the calf. If male, he will probably either be shot and tossed into a bin, or sold to be raised for veal, which delays his death by just a matter of months. But if the calf is female, she will usually be prepared for her own entry into dairy production, where she will face the same cycle of hell that her mother is trapped in: forced impregnation, the theft of her baby, and a return to the cattle crush two or three months later."

David noticed the expression on Peter's face change and suddenly became aware that he'd probably just heard this for the first time. Perhaps he had gone too far.

"I'm sorry if I've shocked you," said David.

"I've always drunk loads of milk, my mother used to give us gallons of the stuff. I had no idea", said Peter.

"*Most* people have no idea," said David. "The dairy industry deliberately hides the truth. And I used to be a part of it! But not only was I beginning to question dairy farming and its morality, but also the wider issues of animal welfare. One evening I was watching TV with the family and there was a short film asking the question, *Why the UK doesn't eat dogs, but people in China do*. They reported that 10,000 dogs would be slaughtered in the annual dog meat festival in Yulin. My daughters were outraged. We have a couple of dogs ourselves and my girls thought that the Chinese must be monsters."

"They do have a point" said Peter.

"Absolutely", said David, "but instead of being outraged by it, I was asking myself whether the actions of the Chinese are any different to what we in the West are doing to pigs, chickens, lambs and cattle".

"There's a huge difference," said Peter defensively. "Pigs and chickens are part of the food chain."

"But the Chinese also believe that dogs are part of the food chain. Who's right?" said David.

"We are, of course. It's obvious," said Peter.

"Well it might be to you and many others, but to me it was becoming less and less obvious why we would keep a dog or a cat as a pet and call ourselves animal lovers while at the same time eating and abusing other defenseless animals for their flesh, milk and skin. Did you know that every year in the UK, approximately 2.6 million cattle, 10 million pigs, 14.5 million sheep and lambs, 80 million fish and 950 million birds are slaughtered for human consumption? That's a lot of suffering."

Of course, Peter had not reached 53 years of age without ever thinking about the meat on his plate. But he'd always believed that the animals had been treated well and that eating meat was normal, necessary and natural. Although David hadn't finished his story, Peter was beginning to question his own worldview. Only yesterday, the nutritionist had effectively told him that it was the meat and dairy that had given him heart disease and that it was perfectly possible and even beneficial to eat plants instead. Here he was now, just a day later, being confronted with the very harsh reality concerning the morality of consuming animals and animal products in the first place.

Suddenly, it all seemed a bit much.

"Bloody hell," Peter muttered. "I only came here for some vegetables for lunch."

"I'm sorry," said David, with a kind smile on his face. "I'll stop now."

Peter almost walked away from the counter then, but he could barely move his trolley, he was so deep in thought. He was becoming aware that a truth that he had held dear for so many years was beginning to crumble. His instincts told him that if he let David continue with his story, it might leave him wrestling with his own conscience. The nutritionist had said it yesterday, too… For the first time since his diagnosis, a glint of something positive entered Peter's mind. What if David's story could in some way help him to overcome his heart disease? And there was something else about David that intrigued Peter; he had an air of peace and calm about him, which - for all Peter's doubts - left him wanting to hear David's story out.

"It's fine," said Peter, "please carry on. It's hard to hear, I'd like to hear more."

David smiled sympathetically, knowingly. He continued.

"Basically, the way I saw the world had changed. Try as I might, there was no more denying it to myself. Then I started thinking about when the next animal transport would be arriving to pick up the next batch of dairy cows that were no longer productive. What was I going to do about it? After all, the farm is a family business and was our only source of income. Meat and dairy farms receive huge subsidies from the government, so it was going to be a challenge to replace that income.

"It was at that point that I decided to talk it through with my wife. I started by explaining to her that - as a first step - I'd decided to become a vegetarian, but that I wanted to move towards a diet that was entirely free of animal products. Then I dropped the bombshell. I told her that I couldn't bring myself to send anymore of our cows to the slaughterhouse. I told her that I'd found an animal sanctuary that would take our remaining cattle and that I wanted to convert the farm into growing organic vegetables. It was a shock, but thankfully my wife was incredibly supportive. Both of us have always had complete faith in each other, so when I told her what I'd been thinking, she was ready to back me up all the way. I love her for that. Having her backing and blessing gave me the strength and determination I needed to see it through."

Peter thought about how supportive Susan had already been since finding out about his heart problems. "I can relate to that", said Peter. "You need backing if you're going to make a massive change like that in your life."

"Absolutely. Once I'd talked in through with my wife and family," David continued, "everything changed for me. I felt as though a heavy weight had been lifted from my shoulders. The day our remaining animals were sent to the sanctuary rather than the slaughterhouse was very special. For years I'd felt pangs of guilt and betrayal and dreaded the lorries arriving. Yet that day symbolized a new start for us and the farm.

That was two years ago. Today, we run an organic farm and as you can see, we've built a shop and café, which have both become very popular with locals," said David.

"I love animals," said Peter. "We have a golden Labrador at home called Sheba."

"Everyone I know loves animals," said David, "but almost everyone I know also loves eating animals. In fact, being strong for animals is relatively easy because you just have to remind people of what they already know. Virtually everyone, unless they are a sociopath, has had the experience of bonding with a dog or a cat. I bet you can't look into your Labrador's eyes without understanding that there is a sentient being behind them. If you were walking down the street and someone started beating a puppy, how long would it take for a crowd to gather and stop them? That's because people are by nature full of kindness and empathy for others and animals. The part of humanity that wants to protect the innocent and defend the vulnerable, that's the best of humanity. Not the part that puts animals in factory farms and eats them," said David.

"But aside from that, rejecting meat and dairy is also so useful in terms of society", he continued, "because when you exercise that empathy towards a voiceless group, it means you're forcing yourself to look beyond your own selfish wants out to the bigger picture and a wider world emerges to you. Animals are voiceless. We need to be the ones to help make the change for them, starting with every time we sit down for a meal.

Peter looked at David.

"That's very thought-provoking. I have heart disease you know. Yesterday, I went to see the nutritionist and she told me that if I want to get better without surgery, I need to cut meat and dairy out of my diet. That's why I'm here."

"Yes, one of the greatest ironies and contradictions of modern society is that the food that we eat is actually making us ill." David laughed. "Making the kind of changes that I've made makes you a bit of an expert and perhaps a bit unpopular."

"To be fair you really know your stuff, or at least you seem to. Do you have an earpiece fitted and someone is telling you what to say", said Peter.

"No", laughed David. "I'm just really passionate about doing what I can to counter the brain washing that we've all endured since being born."

"So you also think that meat and dairy could be to blame for my heart problems", said Peter.

"Well put it like this," said David, "The World Health Organization declared processed meat a carcinogen. Not that processed meat could cause cancer, but that it probably causes colorectal cancer. Another study by Harvard found that one serving a day of red meat in adolescence or early adulthood had a 22% higher risk of breast cancer. Each serving per day led to a 13% higher risk of breast cancer overall. And it isn't just cancer. A Cancer Institute in America did the biggest study ever and linked both processed and unprocessed meat to an increase in death rates from nine diseases. These include heart disease, stroke, diabetes, Alzheimer's and lung disease. So, yes, I think what you were told yesterday has a lot of merit" said David.

"But I'm a farmer, you know, so for me it's more about drawing attention to the animals and their welfare. Have you any idea about the quantities of antibiotics using in farming in the UK and globally?"

"I know antibiotics are used in farming, but I don't know how much", said Peter.

"Well", David said, "Just the other week there was a report from the Foods Standards Agency saying that British supermarket chickens were showing record levels of antibiotic-resistant superbugs. In the US more than 70 percent of antibiotics that are medically important for humans are used in animals.

A lot of the antibiotics are given to healthy animals to prevent infection or speed up their growth. Especially in intensive farming where animals are kept penned in." Crazy, isn't it. We're putting the health of our own children and families at risk in the pursuit of profit."

"To be fair, that does sound risky," said Peter.

"Risky?" said David, "More like utterly stupid. Some last-resort antibiotics for humans are being used a lot in animals and there are no replacements currently on the way. Drug-resistant bugs could be passed on through direct contact between humans and animals, particularly farmers. It's just madness."

"But what's the alternative?" asked Peter.

"What you see right here is my family's vision of a different and more compassionate world", said David. "All of the produce on sale here is organic. We don't grow it all, of course, but we have a reliable supply chain that enables us to offer our customers everything they need to eat in a sustainable way. No animals are hurt or exploited and there's everything you need to create delicious healthy food."

"Sounds like I'm in the right place," said Peter.

"You absolutely are," said David. "In more ways than one".

Peter was realising that his perceptions of meat and dairy farming were rapidly changing thanks to the words and deeds of David, maybe for good. *Yes, probably for good*, he thought to himself. The troublesome part of Peter - the side of him that had denied and deliberately ignored animal welfare and where the meat really came from - did feel a sense of loss. However, the caring, compassionate and humane side of Peter suddenly became energized and empowered. Peter realized that David had just given him the gift of knowledge - knowledge that was so strong and undeniable that it would perhaps help him to achieve his own personal goal of avoiding surgery.

Could it really be true, he thought, *that he had been so wilfully ignorant for his entire life? How could it possibly have taken him 53 years of life to discover something that now seemed blatantly obvious?*

Why has it has taken me until now to grasp what's going on?" Peter said to David, shaking his head in disbelief. "I mean, I'm 53 years old, after all!"

"Don't be so hard on yourself. There are several very strong forces working against our better judgement," David said, "including tradition, culture, politics and lobbying by huge industries. It's a tradition in our culture to eat meat, dairy and eggs and it's a hard habit to break, especially when everyone else is doing it. On top of that, we are bombarded with images, messages, advertising and packaging that promote it as normal, natural and necessary. Just because the tradition and act of eating meat and dairy has been practiced for hundreds and thousands of years does not make it *right*.

"Anyway," David continued, changing the tone, "I can see by the look on your face that you've had enough for now. Please take a look at all the lovely produce that we have here and I hope you'll find some delicious ingredients for your wife."

David made his way to the back of the store, leaving Peter to peruse the aisles. "*Just look at those pears*", Peter thought to himself. He could see that they were perfectly ripe and he picked one up and held it under his nose. *I'll have some of those for Ellie.* Top of his list was lentils and he found them nicely presented on wooden shelving. There were larger lentils and smaller ones, grey lentils, black lentils and even orange and yellow lentils. Peter went for the orange ones. After putting some carrots in his basket, he found the sweet potatoes. One had been cut open to reveal the bright and delicious looking orange interior. There was a sign above them, which read: Sweet Potatoes: *a great source of fiber, vitamins and minerals.* Next up was mushrooms and what a selection. Peter remembered how good mushrooms tasted with onions and garlic. *Don't get carried away and buy too many*, he thought to himself. Just like the sweet potatoes, there was a sign saying

Mushrooms: boost the production of vitamin D, lower cholesterol levels and enhance your immune system. What a fantastic shop this was.

On his way over to the counter to pay he noticed all the alternative plant-based milks on sale. *I've never tried one of those*, thought Peter, and went over to take a look. There was almond milk, rice milk, soy milk, coconut milk, cashew milk, hemp milk and even oat milk. Peter had no idea how they would taste so he just reached for the soy milk because it had the most attractive looking packaging.

Peter paid for his shopping, told David that it had been a pleasure to meet him and made his way out of the store to head back home.

Everyone was out when he got home, apart from Sheba, the Labrador, who greeted him wagging her tail ferociously in delight at his arrival.. He made himself a cup of tea and sat down on the sofa with a biscuit. He wondered whether the biscuit contained milk. He laughed to himself, aware that it was the first time he'd asked himself such a question. Sheba was sitting patiently a couple of paces away from him with her eyes fixed in a laser-like manner on the biscuit that Peter was about to put in his mouth. He looked at Sheba, she looked at him and then back to the biscuit and back to Peter again. They had played this scene out many times in the past and she knew he would surrender and share his biscuit. He liked to keep her in suspense, but he always gave her a bite. He loved Sheba.

What does all this mean? thought Peter. He went through it all slowly in his mind. *I'm a married man with two daughters and a loving wife. I'm a van driver at the post office. I like my job because it's simple and steady. I have heart disease and they've said I need an operation. Yesterday, I met Gail, the nutritionist who told me there might be another way for me to return to health without surgery. I've just got back from the farmer who has told me about the horrors and cruelty of meat and dairy farming, which further supports the direction the nutritionist was recommending. And Michael and Gail told me that I need a goal as well. Apparently, I need some motivation over and above wanting to get well again. So what makes me feel really alive and energized? What one change could make my life happier? What did I used to love doing as a kid?*

Just then the door opened. It was Susan and Ellie.

"Did you get the ingredients, Peter?" Susan asked.

"I did and I got some soya milk for us to try". "Yuck", said Ellie, "that sounds horrible.

"Well you'll never know unless you try it", said Peter.

"Dad," said Ellie, "Mum says you can take me to get the shower heads this afternoon."

"Did she?" replied Peter. "OK, we'll go together this afternoon. Satisfied now?"

"Yes, it'll do."

CHAPTER 6 : THE ENVIRONMENTALIST

ater that afternoon, Peter and Ellie went to the hardware superstore to get the low-flow shower heads that Ellie had been banging on about for days.

"So just remind me," said Peter, "why are we getting these?"

"Because we'll use less hot water, which saves energy," Ellie replied. "And we'll use less water, which is also good."

The store was huge, so they followed the signage for the plumbing supplies area. As they both turned into the isle, they saw a young woman stacking the shelves.

"Excuse me," said Peter, "we're looking for the low-flow shower heads."

"Yes," interrupted Ellie, "we're going to help prevent climate change."

"With a shower head? I don't think so," said the woman. "That's all but useless, like throwing a baked bean at an Elephant. If you really want to do something for the environment and help to stop climate change, it's up to us, the younger generation, to actively do something to reverse the damage that we're causing."

"Like what?" said Ellie, instantly interested in the woman's words.

"Tell you what, I don't see any harm in telling you, although don't clue in my manager! Probably shouldn't be talking about this during work hours, but there's a meeting this evening in St. Thomas's Church Hall and it's all about climate change. I'm studying about environmental issues at uni, you see. There's a world-renowned expert coming to talk about the environment and the one change anyone can make that will effectively halve your carbon footprint. My top tip for you is save your money and go to the free meeting instead, I've been told it will blow your mind!"

"Can we go, Dad?" said Ellie.

"I thought you wanted a shower head," said Peter.

"Please? I want to go to the meeting instead now!"

"What time does it start, er – I didn't catch your name?" asked Peter.

"I'm Lea," the woman replied, smiling. "It starts at 7 and it will last about an hour and a half."

"Alright then," said Peter, reluctantly. "We can go after dinner and after your mum and I have taken the dog for a walk."

"I'll be there, too," said Lea, "So I'll see you tonight then!"

Susan, Ellie and Peter usually took it in turns to take Sheba the dog for a walk. But this evening, Peter invited Susan to come with him so that he could share all that David had told him at the farm shop earlier. There is something about going for a walk that changes the dynamic of a conversation; it somehow feels like you are both going in the same direction. This is what Peter wanted with Susan; he'd made up his mind to stop eating all animal products, both for his own health *and* for the sake of the animals. Strangely enough, he'd only committed to making this profound change in his life this morning, just a few hours ago, and yet he was already feeling better about himself.

"So the farm guy basically turned you into tree-hugging, animal lover?" Susan laughed as they walked along the path.

"I've always been an animal lover!" replied Peter. "But honestly, it was inspiring to hear him talk about how he used to farm the animals and send them away for slaughter for a living, something that his family had been doing for years. Then he really put his ethics and conscience first. I hope it works out for him. Before you got back earlier, I had a cup of tea with Sheba and the penny finally dropped. I need to make a change in my life. What do you think?"

"Well," said Susan, "we could try and do it together. I'm up for it if you are?"

Peter knew that getting Susan's support would be crucial to being successful. He might be able to let himself down, but he would find it more difficult to let Susan down.

Peter and Ellie arrived at five to seven at the Church Hall. There was a sign saying, *You can make a big difference. Free entrance if you're open to change.* As they walked in Peter became aware of that musty smell that all churches seem to have. Around 100 chairs had been put out and the hall it was already around two-thirds full. There was a platform at the front that had been raised just a few inches from the floor. There was no microphone.

"Hello," said a voice from behind. They turned to find Lea beaming at them. "You came, then!"

"Well, you said it would blow our minds, so here we are," replied Peter.

"It's just about to start," said Lea. "Let's see what we can learn."

At 7 pm sharp, a sharply-dressed woman of around 40-years of age walked out from the side and took her place on the stage. She made a calm, relaxed and confident impression on Peter.

"Good evening ladies and gentlemen. My name is Joanne and it's nice to see you all here this evening. I'm going to jump right into it, because I know from experience that time flies and there's a dance class at 8.30, so we can't overrun. But I'd just like to say that hopefully this evening you'll learn some striking facts about the environment and climate change. You'll also learn about step that you can make to offset your own impact on the planet. If what you learn resonates with you, please spread the word. I believe that we all have the power to make a difference"

Peter thought it was weird that he found himself sitting here. This would be the third time the matter of only a few days that he found himself listening and learning new facts about problems that he had always known existed. He laughed to himself has he sat up straight in his chair and thought *It's like buses, you wait for ages and then three come at once.*

Joanne cleared her throat.

"The earth is home to us all. We all have a vested interested in looking after our planet. We have all heard about climate change and the environmental damage that humankind is inflicting on Planet Earth. This evening you're going to hear things you might already know and many things that you don't. But the good news is that you are all going to be empowered by the time you leave this hall this evening. You're going to learn how you can slash your carbon footprint in half – yes, that's right, by a whopping 50 percent - by making *one* change in your lives. Not only will this change cost you absolutely nothing, it will probably also save you money and leave you and your family healthier and happier.

"But before I address the practical things we can all do, I think it's fitting to briefly summarize the adverse impact that we are having on our planet. First and perhaps the most well-known impact is climate change. According to NASA, global climate change has already had observable effects on the environment. Glaciers have shrunk, ice on rivers and lakes is breaking up earlier, plant and animal ranges have shifted, and trees are flowering sooner. Effects that scientists had predicted in the past would result from global climate change are now occurring: loss of sea ice, accelerated sea level rise and longer, more intense heat waves.

"Scientists have high confidence that global temperatures will continue to rise for decades to come, largely due to greenhouse gases produced by human activities. Temperatures will continue to rise, the frost-free season will lengthen, there will be changes in precipitation patterns, more droughts and heat waves, hurricanes will become stronger and more intense, global sea level will rise by 1-4 feet by 2100 and the arctic is likely to become ice free.

"But in addition to climate change, other major global problems include water use or rather clean water shortages, waste - I'm sure we've all heard about the huge damage that plastic is doing - land use, dead zones in our oceans, species extinction and deforestation.

"However," said Joanne, "as I mentioned, my intention this evening is not to add to any feeling of helplessness that you may have, but instead to empower you all. I'd like to ask a question. What do you think is the 'single biggest way' to reduce your impact on Earth and the environment?"

The audience sat quietly for a moment before a man on the left said, "getting rid of our cars"

"Well, that would make a difference, but it's by no means the most important."

A woman sitting next to him said, "insulating our homes"

"Again, it would make a difference, but it's far overshadowed by another behaviour that we all do several times a day."

Peter had remained quiet; he was sitting and listening with great interest. When Joanne had asked the question, his first thought had been his car, too. But then he started to think, *it couldn't be that as well, could it?* He'd heard about the damage that meat had done to his health yesterday, this morning he'd learned about the cruelty of eating animals, and now he was sitting on the edge of his seat about to shout it out as a suggestion.

"Is it eating meat?" said Peter loudly, so that everyone could hear.

"Thank you," said Joanne, "that's exactly right - or more specifically meat, dairy and all animal products. Animal Agriculture is the most destructive industry facing the planet today. There is a film, which I recommend that you all watch, called *Cowspiracy*. The film's makers put together some shocking facts, here are just some of them."

Joanne changed the slide on the screen, reading the listed facts aloud and adding to them as she spoke to the listening crowd:

- Livestock and their byproducts account for at least 32,000 million tons of carbon dioxide (CO2) per year, or 51% of all worldwide greenhouse gas emissions.
- Livestock is responsible for 65% of all human-related emissions of nitrous oxide – a greenhouse gas with 296 times the global warming potential of carbon dioxide, and which stays in the atmosphere for 150 years.
- Even without fossil fuels, we will exceed our 565 gigatonnes CO2e limit by 2030, all from raising animals.
- 2,500 gallons of water are needed to produce 1 pound of beef.
- 477 gallons of water are required to produce 1lb. of eggs; almost 900 gallons of water are needed for 1lb. of cheese.
- 5% of water consumed in the US is by private homes. 55% of water consumed in the US is for animal agriculture.
- Animal agriculture is the leading cause of species extinction, ocean dead zones, water pollution, and habitat destruction. Animal agriculture contributes to species extinction in many ways. In addition to the monumental habitat destruction caused by clearing forests and converting land to grow feed crops and for animal grazing, predators and "competition" species are frequently targeted and hunted because of a perceived threat to livestock profits.
- The widespread use of pesticides, herbicides and chemical fertilizers used in the production of feed crops often interferes with the reproductive systems of animals and poison waterways. The overexploitation of wild species through commercial fishing, bushmeat trade as well as animal agriculture's impact on climate change, all contribute to global depletion of species and resources.
- Livestock operations on land have created more than 500 nitrogen flooded dead zones around the world in our oceans.
- A farm with 2,500 dairy cows produces the same amount of waste as a city of 411,000 people.

- 130 times more animal waste than human waste is produced in the US – 1.4 billion tons from the meat industry annually. 5 tons of animal waste is produced per person in the US.
- 3/4 of the world's fisheries are exploited or depleted.
- As many as 2.7 trillion animals are pulled from the ocean each year.
- For every 1 pound of fish caught, up to 5 pounds of unintended marine species are caught and discarded as by-kill.
- Animal agriculture is responsible for up to 91% of Amazonian forest destruction.
- Up to 137 plant, animal and insect species are lost every day due to rainforest destruction.
- Ten thousand years ago, 99% of biomass (i.e. zoomass) was wild animals. Today, humans and the animals that we raise as food make up 98% of the zoomass.
- 70% of antibiotic sold in the US are for livestock.
- 70 billion farmed animals are reared annually worldwide. More than 6 million animals are killed for food every hour.
- Throughout the world, humans drink 5.2 billion gallons of water and eat 21 billion pounds of food each day. Compare that with Worldwide, cows drink 45 billion gallons of water and eat 135 billion pounds of food each day.
- 82% of starving children live in countries where food is fed to animals, and the animals are eaten by western countries.
- Land required to feed 1 person for 1 year: Vegan: 1/6th acre, Vegetarian: 3x as much as a vegan, Meat Eater: 18x as much as a vegan
- A person who follows a vegan diet produces the equivalent of 50% less carbon dioxide, uses 1/11th oil, 1/13th water, and 1/18th land compared to a meat-lover for their food.
- Each day, a person who eats a vegan diet saves 1,100 gallons of water, 45 pounds of grain, 30 sq ft of forested land, 20 lbs CO2 equivalent, and one animal's life.

Joanne finished reading out her list and paused. Peter, like everyone else in the room sat quietly taking in the information that had just been shared with them. Lea the student had promised Peter earlier that the speech this evening would blow their minds, and she was right. Speaking to the farmer earlier, Peter recognized that he'd felt uncomfortable deep down for many years about eating animals. In a way, he had been aware on some level, but had chosen to ignore the signals because eating meat, fish and dairy was what he and everyone he knew did. Put simply, it was part of tradition and culture.

But this was different. In his mind, Peter had never contemplated the environmental costs of eating meat and dairy when compared to a plant-based diet. If what Joanne was saying was true, it was truly shocking. Yet for all the horrors of what he had just been told there was something that, at this very moment, felt even more scandalous. *Why* had he never been told and *why* had it taken being diagnosed with heart disease for him to find out?

"They didn't tell us that at school," whispered Ellie.

Peter replied, "They never told us either."

"Before I go on", said Joanne, "are there any questions?"

Ellie put up her hand and Joanne gestured for her to speak.

"We've been doing a school project on climate change and the environment for the past two weeks. None of this was mentioned."

Joanne replied, "That's not surprising. I think the main problem is that most teachers, educators and policy makers are all meat eaters. It's difficult to highlight the problems of eating meat and dairy and advocate giving it up when you yourself eat the stuff. That would be hypocritical. Actually, there is a short story from the past and from the tobacco industry that explains this perfectly.

Scientists in the USA established the first links between smoking and cancer as early as the 1930s. Yet even in the 1950s, the American Medical Association was still saying that, on balance, smoking is good for you! None of the hundreds and later thousands of studies showing the harmful effects of smoking made it out into the public realm. The average American smoked at least a half pack of cigarettes a day, including doctors, the government, the medical community, everyone. Even though there was an unassailable body of evidence linking smoking to cancer, it was kept quiet simply because smoking was what everyone did. In the end it took no less than 7000 studies linking smoking to cancer before the Surgeon General's report in 1964 finally said there was a relationship between smoking cigarettes and dangerous health effects, including lung cancer and heart disease."

Joanne looked around the room.

"What's happening today is just the same", she continued. "There is clear evidence that the single most important step that each and everyone of us can take to help the environment is to stop eating meat and dairy. The government could also start getting serious by phasing out subsidies to the meat and dairy industries. If consumers had to pay the true price of meat and dairy, much less of it would be consumed. How can it be that a litre of milk cost less than a litre of water in the UK and most of the EU? Because of *subsidies*, of course, and this also applies to meat and dairy. It's scandalous", said Joanne.

A hand from the audience was raised. A man who Peter thought looked in his late 50s made a statement.

"There's a big problem with your solution, I'm afraid," he said. "People just don't want to change. You might be able to persuade them to change a light bulb or something, but there's no way they are going to give up meat and dairy. You'd be lucky to even get people to cut down a little bit. People are actually addicted to cheese and meat. I've been eating a plant-based diet for nearly 20 years and I've completely given up on any hope that people will change their ways. They just won't. You're right to point out to people the impact of animal agriculture on the environment, because I do think that change starts with awareness. But it's not the solution, because its impractical in the minds of the vast majority. My suggestion would be that people start to cut down or do a meat-free Monday or something.

Have you ever heard of clean meat?"

"Yes, that's an excellent point, said Joanne. For those of you who don't know clean meat is basically meat that is grown in a lab. It's meat without the animal, it looks like meat and tastes like meat simply because it is meat. But it produces 96 percent fewer emissions, is free from growth hormones, antibiotics and no animals are killed."

"But unlike agriculture, there's no government funding", the man in the audience said.

"I know, Joanne said, "we still have a long way to go, but progress is being made. As far as I'm aware, it's purely private investment that's fuelling the research and development of clean meat at the moment and we certainly need to get the government on board, but there is a lot of resistance. There was a study that showed that many people find the thought of cultured meat disgusting and wouldn't want to eat it. There is also a large number of powerful groups that are working against any challenge to the meat and dairy industries. These groups have a very strong political lobby.

You say that people will never change their eating habits," Joanne continued, "but I think we are witnessing a change in our culture. The number of people eating a purely plant-based diet has surged by 700 percent in just two years. 14 percent of Britain's population - more than 7 million people - are now vegetarian. A more 'environmentally conscious public' is also said to be behind the changes in the UK, as awareness surrounding the sustainability of animal products continues to grow. So there *is* hope."

"If I may," said Joanne summing up, "I'd like to leave you with this thought. The next time you hear people on the TV or radio explaining that we should drive more fuel-efficient cars, or that we should use less water, ride our bikes more or change our light bulbs, remember that all of these things pale into insignificance by comparison to reducing or cutting out completely meat and dairy from your diet. It's the single most effective and selfless act you can make for the good of the planet and the plants and animals that we share this unique world with.

Save the Planet. Eat Plants.

Thank you."

"Well," said Peter as he and Ellie made their way out of the Church Hall, "it's been a very interesting day."

Ellie nodded, deep in thought herself.

Peter couldn't help but consider the events of the past few days, about meeting Gail the nutritionist, David at the farm, and now listening to the words of Joanne here tonight.

Back at home, he took his next dose of aspirin before bed - he'd been taking it exactly as he'd been prescribed and he *was* feeling better. Earlier that afternoon, he'd called in to work; they had asked him if he could continue if he felt up to it and wanted to. *Did* he want to? Surely, the worst thing he could do would be to hang around at home, mulling over his condition and what the future held for him. No, he decided to go back to work. He would just have to take things slowly.

CHAPTER 7 : THE LADS

It was Friday night and Peter decided to go out with the lads despite his illness and worries. He thought a night out might cheer him up. Peter's friends had been his rock for so long, he couldn't remember a problem he hadn't talked to them about, usually over a beer. They were there for him over a round of golf when he was working up the courage to ask out Susan. When one their group and close friend of Peter had died suddenly, they'd had Friday night drink in his honour. But what would they say now? Surely they would pity him when he talked about his heart diagnosis. Then again, they would almost certainly make a few jokes at his expense. But that was fine for Peter because it was all well intentioned. What would they say about what he'd learnt over the past few days? Between the nutritionist, the farmer, and the environmentalist, he'd had a real change of heart. Would they see it his way, too?

They'd arranged to meet at 8 pm and Peter got there five minutes early. Two of his friends were already there wearing a smile and holding a pint of larger.

"Ey up," said Peter, greeting his mates before making his way to the bar to get himself a pint. By 8.30 the group had grown to eight and the next round of drinks were already being ordered.

"Have you heard?" said Martin. "There's been a theft at the Viagra factory. The police are looking for some hardened criminals!"

They'd started.

Peter said, "I think I might have to go and get some of the over-the-counter Viagra myself." His mates, of course, wanted more details. "I can't get it up anymore", he said. "It's been a bit tricky for ages, but the other night it was complete failure."

Dave nudged him with glee. "Impotence. It's nature's way of saying, 'no hard feelings'!"

Jeff laughed heartily as Martin chimed in.

"I've heard that eating Brazil nuts and one vegan meal a day can help you out in that department."

"Bollocks. Just go to the chemists, Peter, it's much easier. That's what I do," said Chris.

"Well," said Peter, "it might not be that easy. You see it's not just that, I've got other problems too. I had a turn at work a few days ago. I've found out that I've got heart disease and they've told me a need a heart bypass."

As he'd expected his mates were sympathetic and encouraging. Peter explained that he wasn't sure about the bypass surgery, and told them more about what he'd learned. He tentatively said that he was thinking of trying out the plant-based option and exercise instead, but that he'd not make a final decision yet.

"And if what you say is true about the brazil nuts, Martin," said Peter, "it might even help with my sex life and cost a lot less than Viagra!" Simon piped up, "that sounds like a right load of rubbish. This nutritionist woman sounds like a hippy. Does she talk a lot about energy vibrations and the like?"

They all laughed.

"It's not just her," said Peter. "There's this Michael bloke at Susan's yoga class…"

Peter told them all about Michael, running marathons and training for an Iron Man despite being diagnosed with heart disease three years ago.

"It all sounds dodgy to me," said Simon. "You'll never stick to fruit and vegetables. I'll give you a week at the most. I don't think I could stop eating meat, I like the taste of it too much, and I'll tell you something else. I think you've been brainwashed by this nutritionist you've been to see. I bet she's a vegan and just wants everyone to eat tasteless, boring food. Well I say that eating animals is natural."

But then Richard, who had been quietly listening, spoke up. "Natural, are you sure about that? Could you kill an animal and eat it? I mean, if someone walked in here with a cow right now, first of all would you feel hungry, and secondly could you kill it to eat?"

"How many beers have you had", replied Simon, "I just don't see any logic in what you're saying. You just go to the supermarket and buy meat fresh from the shelf. Anyway, I didn't realize you were a closet vegan. Are you outing yourself?", he said laughing.

"I'm not", replied Richard, "but you said eating animals is natural."

"It is", said Simon defensively.

"But if you think about it, we would all be hopeless at trying to catch and kill an animal. We weren't given any natural tools for running down and killing an animal. Just imagine trying to catch a rabbit, you'd die first for sure".

"Maybe were natural scavengers then", said Simon, "perhaps we're meant to roam the plains of Africa and eat the leftovers from kills made by other animals".

Richard said, "so you'd eat all the innards, too".

"Of course he wouldn't" said Jeff, "and neither would I because it puts me off my food."

Richard said "But if eating animals is natural, surely you would love and eat all the innards and everything, just like a lion does. And you've still not told us if you could kill a cow. I know couldn't. Better still, if someone walked in here with a lamb, could you slit it's throat and then chop off its leg for a to make a delicious lamb shank"?

"I'm sorry Rich, but you're talking absolute rubbish." Said Simon "That's not how it works, we live in the 21st century and people don't roam round killing animals like that. It's all done humanely in a slaughterhouse. I need another drink to cope with Rich tonight. Where are you getting all this from mate?"

"I'll tell you later, said Richard, but did you know that the definition of the word humane is "having or showing compassion or benevolence. Which means that the word humane and shooting animals are not compatible."

"Come on Rich out with it", said Jeff, "who's been getting into you head". "My daughter", replied Richard", "she's been vegetarian for a few years and a year or so ago she went vegan. I'm not yet, but she has some very powerful arguments."

Simon returned from the bar with another round of drinks. Peter who had remained silent during the exchanges took a second beer from Simon and said thanks.

"Well I say you only live once and I certainly intend to enjoy this beer, but also the delicious taste of meat. You have to admit that vegan food is absolutely tasteless", said Simon.

"Really", said Richard", that beer in your hand is vegan, is it tasteless"?

"No, it's delicious and listening to you tonight I think I'm going to need a few more." They all laughed.

Richard spoke again "This is fun, I think I've got you all a little rattled."

Peter decided to speak up, too "the nutritionist told me that most of the food that we eat is already vegan, things like fruit, vegetables, rice, beans, nuts, seeds, pasta, bread, potatoes and oats."

"But what about bacon", said Simon, "that's not on her list".

"Just because it tastes nice, does not make it morally acceptable", said Richard with a friendly smile on his face. "Surely tormenting and slaughtering a defenceless animal just to have a brief nice taste in your mouth is wrong?"

"There you are", said Simon, "these vegans types go around judging others and that's why everyone hates them."

Richard replied, "I'm not vegan, but my daughter would say that you're being defensive because deep down you know it's wrong to eat meat. She'd say that vegans are just rational human beings who are capable of making a distinction between right and wrong, good and bad, selfish and benevolent". Think of this, Simon, said Richard. "If you were walking down the street and you saw a man butchering a puppy, how would you react?"

"To be honest, I'd be shocked and would probably intervene", said Simon.

"Would you judge him?", asked Richard, "if he said that he was doing it because he loved the taste of puppy meat and wanted to make a sandwich out of it later that evening to enjoy while watching the football on telly, would that be OK with you".

"That's completely different", said Simon, "dogs are pets, and nobody eats dogs. They probably don't even taste nice."

Peter remembered what the David the farmer had told him about the annual dog festival in China. "They eat dogs in China, South Korea, Vietnam and Nigeria", said Peter, "The farmer told me only the other day."

Darren had also been listening to the backwards and forwards of the debate. He was wondering what had happened to the usual banter about football and women, when a thought crossed his mind. "If we didn't eat animals, there wouldn't be enough food for everyone", he said.

"Exactly", said Simon.

Richard weighed in again, "I'm sorry lads, I tried that one at home too on my daughter, but as an argument for eating meat it's about as much use as a chocolate fireguard. What you're basically saying,

Darren, is that if you couldn't eat a cow, you would eat more corn than the cow you would otherwise have eaten. I didn't realize either but feeding cows to then eat them is really inefficient. If the world stopped eating meat it would free up huge areas of land and, apparently, it would stop deforestation in the Amazon as well.

Darren said "Oh, well, it was just a thought and here's another one, can we just talk about football like we usually do?"

Now it was Jeff's turn to speak up, "No, wait, I think this is important, our mate Peter here is on the verge of changing everything and we are his closest and most respected advisors", he said laughing out loud. "The advice that we give him tonight could make all the difference. It's clearly serious, because he's thinking of becoming a vegan!"

Peter explained that he was thinking of becoming vegan primarily for the sake of his health in the hope that he could avoid surgery.

"Well", said Simon, who was turning out to be the strongest advocate for eating meat, "I'd be very wary of anyone telling me that eating just plants is going to make you healthy. For one, where are you going to get your protein?"

"Arnold Schwarzenegger is a vegan you know", said Richard.

"Oh no, not you again Rich, Sheffield's leading authority on a pant-based lifestyle, said Simon.

"I'm only playing Devil's advocate and sharing some myth-busting facts with you, said Richard. "Carl Lewis, Mike Tyson and Novak Djokovic are also vegan. I mean, to win Wimbledon against Federer, he must be getting enough protein. And to just gently bring us all back into our comfort zone of talking about football, Lionel Messi and Sergio Aguero are also vegan, and there from Argentina for god's sake, where meat is the national religion."

"Well I'm not going to change my mind", said Simon, "I think Vegans are extreme".

"Until just a few days ago, I thought the same as you Simon", said Peter, I thought vegans were extremists. Now I'm not so sure".

Richard, who was clearly enjoying himself in his new-found role of Devil's advocate, said "I think vegans seem extreme because it's not the norm. But if you asked a vegan, they would probably think that killing and eating animals without necessity seems extreme."

"Are you all deaf", said Simon, that's my whole point. Eating meat is necessary!"

"But I thought we'd just discovered that it's not", said Richard. "There are millions of vegans from all walks of life that are clearly healthy, including Sergio Aguero".

"Humans are superior to animals", said Simon.

"We're not superior in our ability to fly or see in the dark", said Jeff, who now also seemed happy to weigh in on the side of the animals. "Surely superiority doesn't give us the right to abuse harmless sentient beings?"

"To be fair, said Darren, "I agree with Simon, demanding more rights for animals is only a short step away from claiming they should also have the right to vote."

"Saying that animals should have the right to vote is just silly", said Richard, "but surely it does make sense to give them the right to life?".

"What about plants, then", said Simon, "surely, they have the right to life too and who knows, maybe plants feel pain?".

"Are you really suggesting that digging up a carrot and eating it is the same as killing a dog?", said Richard. "Plants don't have brains or a central nervous system. And, anyway, Simon, even if plants did feel pain, it would still make sense to eat less animals because animals are the ones that are eating most of the plants in the first place."

Peter was very surprised by the passion that his mates had adopted around the subject of eating meat. Clearly what people ate was very personal and closely tied up with their identity and feeling of self. Peter could see that despite the light-hearted way in which he put forward his arguments, Simon was resolute in his beliefs about eating meat. Peter reflected on his own feelings. Listening to his friends, he was beginning to wonder whether a paradigm that society had held so dear for so long was beginning to crumble. While Peter had hoped he would get support from his friends, he'd not expected them to consider all the arguments with such vigour.

"Could you kill an animal, Simon?", said Peter.

They all went quiet and waited for Simon to reply.

"If was alone on a desert island and I need to survive, yes I could", replied Simon.

"That's a cop-out, said Richard, "Could you kill a pig right now so that you could enjoy a bacon sandwich later?".

Simon said, "No, probably not, but I still insist that you're only here once and I want to enjoy myself. Anyway, everyone eats meat and it's only a few extremists that have to get all moral and judgemental and look down on everyone else. I enjoy meat, if you don't then go ahead and become a vegan."

"Do you think that vegans don't enjoy eating meat and cheese?", said Richard.

"Well they can't do, otherwise they wouldn't give it up.", replied Simon.

"Maybe they have more self-control and mental resilience than your typical meat eater, said Richard, "to be honest, it sounds to me as though your addicted, Simon.

Peter said, "Well I love a bacon sandwich and don't get me started on cheese on toast, but I'm thinking of giving it up to get healthy again anyway."

"There you are", said Simon, "we're right back where we started." "There's nothing as tasty as a bacon sandwich and that's why I say that you'll never stick to it. And that's why I say that these vegan types cannot like eating meat, because otherwise they'd never stick to a boring and tasteless diet".

"My plan is to start finding out how to cook tasty meals made out of plants", said Peter, I'm hoping that with time, my diet will be just as tasty as yours, Simon, but without all the cholesterol that's bunged up my arteries.".

"Good for you, Pete", said Richard "Go for it, and now that Simon has laid down the gauntlet by doubting you, you probably have a better chance of sticking to it than before."

Then Simon spoke up again, "What about you then, Rich, you've been spouting off about all the virtues of going vegan, are you still eating meat?"

"Yes, but….",

Richard didn't have time to finish because Simon interrupted, "I can't believe it, you've been standing here for the last half an hour contradicting everything I say you're still eating meat yourself".

"Well, Simon", said Richard, "if you'll just let me finish. I was going to say that I've managed to cut down quite a bit, but I'm still struggling to kick my bacon and cheese addiction."

Jeff asked, "Do you want to cut meat and dairy out altogether Richard"

"Yes", said Richard

"Why", asked Jeff?

Peter had also been wondering where Richard had got all the information and had been surprised by his revelation that he was trying to go plant-based.

Richard said, "I told you all earlier, it's my daughter. Basically, she went vegetarian a few years ago. I thought it was just a fad and didn't think too much about it. But then, one evening about a year ago, she told us all that she was going to go vegan. I was horrified and I actually had this vision of a weak and pale daughter who would wither away in front of me." Richard started to laugh. "I asked her the classic question, the question that could only come from someone with absolutely no idea and complete ignorance. I asked, where are you going to get your protein?".

"That was my question to the nutritionist", said Peter agreeing.

Richard continued, "she assured me that if I looked it up, I would find out that there is protein in lots of plants and that I didn't have to worry. Do you know what she said to me, it really made me sit up and think. She said that when you open our fridge door it looks like a morgue; full of body parts of dead animals. I'm not sure why, but that really struck a chord in me. She said that when we opened the fridge it should be full of colour and contain fresh things provided by nature. Over the past months I've been slowly finding out what this vegan and plant-based thing is all about and as you can probably tell from tonight, I've picked up quite a lot."

"You're not kidding, there", said Jeff, "Your performance this evening could have been from someone with an honours degree on the subject."

"She's persistent", said Richard, proudly."

"That's weird about the fridge", said Jeff, "I've never heard that before". "Sounds like the contents of my fridge, too, to be honest."

Darren said, "If you ask me, you're all doing it wrong, a fridge should be full of beer and nothing else." They all laughed. Then Darren continued, "I know it's been fascinating going on about food and what you can eat and what you can't eat, but can we change the subject because if I listen much longer, I might start to get a guilty conscience about what I eat. And after all, whatever is wrong with just eating a balanced diet and not getting too extreme one way or the other."

Peter said, "but the question is, what is a balanced diet? I mean, I've just been diagnosed with heart disease and for years and years I thought I was eating a relatively healthy balanced diet."

Simon said, "it's probably in your genes Peter, all this going vegan rubbish is not going to help you. Did the heart doctor mention your diet?"

"No", said Peter.

"I rest my case." said Simon.

"So you don't think diet has anything do to with my heart disease?", said Peter.

"Nope", said Simon. "Personally, I'd rather have the OP than give up all my favourite foods. I think you're clutching at straws".

"Wow" said Peter. "That's the opposite of what I've started thinking."

Strangely, listening to Simon's arguments this evening seemed to confirm what the nutritionist had told him about the majority of people being unwilling to make changes in their lives for the sake of their health.

Richard said, "take no notice of him, Pete, if I were you, I'd definitely give going plant-based a try. As I see it you've nothing to lose and everything to gain."

Simon said, "of course he's got something to lose, his quality of life!

Richard said, "well just maybe, Simon, Pete's quality of life is defined by more than a bacon sandwich!

Thanks to my daughter, the contents of our fridge have transformed over the past year. And I've discovered that actually, it can be really delicious."

Richard continued, I'm almost at the point where I don't really need to eat meat anymore.

"Cheers, Richard," said Peter. "I was hoping that one of you Neanderthals would back me up and give me some encouragement."

"Hey, I've got something for you Peter", said Darren, "me and Russel can back you up, too, but in a different way."

"Go on", said Peter.

"Why don't you come with us on Sunday?" said Darren. "Me and Russ are going out into the Peak District for a bit of walking, hiking and that. We're going to finish with a pint in the pub."

Peter and all his mates used to drive out to the Peak District when they were in their late teens and early twenties, just after they had all passed their driving tests and got their first cars. It was only just east from Sheffield, rocky and bare, but also beautiful and boasting plenty of spectacular walks. Peter found the suggestion very appealing. He used to love going out on the hills for a walk, but it had been years since he last went out there.

"We're going to start going out every weekend and want to make it into a regular thing," said Darren. Then he laughed. "We like the idea of having a good bracing walk followed by a pint in a countryside pub as a reward."

Suddenly, Peter was hit by a surge of motivation. This was it! He would give this plant-based diet and exercise thing a chance, because his objective could be to join the lads on a Sunday morning for a hike in the Peak District.

"I would love to come, Darren," said Peter, "but I'm not up to it at the moment. Those chest pains I got at work the other day were only from trying to carry two sacks down a couple of flights of stairs. I don't think it would be a good idea to come this weekend. But, I'll tell you what, I'm going to start on this diet the nutritionist told me about and I'm going to get fit again. I've decided right now over this pint of beer to call off the operation. As soon as I can, I'm going to be joining you on Sundays for a hike. I've been told I needed a goal and now I have one. Fantastic. Cheers lads!

Peter had always walked home after meeting up with his friends. It only took 15 minutes and he'd decided to stick to old habits tonight despite his heart problem. He'd just take it nice and slowly. Normally, he'd go to the fish and chip shop and get something to eat while he was walking home. But tonight, he decided to go without. He reflected on the evening. They had been meeting up on a Friday night for years and years, and yet tonight had been one of the strangest he'd ever had. Darren was right, they usually talked about football, women or utter nonsense, it was just a laugh really.

As he walked home, he thought about telling Susan about all that had been said in the pub. She knew all his friends and Peter knew that she would be as surprised as he was when he told her. Simon also crossed his mind again. Peter had been surprised about how defensive he'd been and hadn't expected him to react so strongly. Food was something that obviously meant a great deal to Simon in terms of defining who he was.

Peter reached home and Sheba the dog let out a couple of weak barks from inside. As he opened the door, she greeted him with her tail wagging, her head lowered and a great show of affection as usual. "I can't believe people eat dogs in China, he thought to himself sadly."

Everything was changing.!"

CHAPTER 8 : PUTTING CHANGE INTO ACTION

It was Monday morning and Peter was back in the kitchen. Over the weekend, he'd been thinking more about changing his diet and getting started with exercise. He'd started by considering his current diet, the one that had seemingly led him to angina and heart disease. Virtually all his meals currently included meat or fish. Cheese was another one of his favourites. Most of his thoughts focused on what he'd no longer be able to eat, and when he mentally went through his typical meals and cut out the meat and dairy there wasn't a lot left. Then there were his regular treats: chocolate bars, cake, ice cream and the like. These *all* contained milk or dairy, so presumably these would also be off the menu as far as Peter was concerned.

He'd used the weekend to browse the internet in an attempt to find solid information about what he should be eating and how he should be exercising. If anything, it had left him more confused than before. The sheer volume of advice, opinion and data had left him overwhelmed and confused, not least because much of it seemed contradictory. He'd decided to go back to see the nutritionist, Gail, to get a solid diet and exercise plan. After all, she was the one who'd started him down this track so it seemed only logical to seek her advice again.

"Dad," said Ellie over the breakfast table. "Do you think that woman was telling the truth about the environment at that meeting we went to? It's the last day of our project today and we're going to be summarizing everything we've learned. Do you think I should mention all the destruction that the animals are doing and that it's really our own fault for eating them?"

"What do you think?" said Peter. "What do you want to do?"

"They've not told us anything about the damage we are causing by eating all these animal products, so I think I'm going to mention it and see what they say. It's not the teachers, I don't care what they say. It's how my friends and the other kids will react, that's all."

"So," said Susan as she joined them, "what's for breakfast?"

"I've no idea, really," Peter replied. "I've just looked in the cupboard and fridge and everything has got milk or meat in it. So I'm going to have dry toast, I think that should be OK"

"Dry toast?" said Susan, obviously aghast.

"I know," said Peter, "but I'm going to sort it all out today. I've got another appointment to see Gail, so I'm going to ask her for a diet plan and some practical advice on what to buy and how to transition. I love my food. I want to enjoy eating and drinking just as much as I do at the moment.

"I'm sure Gail will be able to point you in the right direction," Susan said. "No more dry toast for breakfast!"

"Absolutely! I'm trying to keep positive and force my mind to believe that there might be a world where it's possible to eat only plants and still enjoy your food. I'll be here this evening when you get back – hopefully I'll be a step further!"

That morning, Gail smiled as Peter walked in through the door.

"Nice to see you again," she said. "How are you feeling?"

"Less confused than a few days ago," Peter confessed, "but I need some direction, because at the moment I'm only eating dried toast for breakfast and I'm not impressed. I want to give myself a chance with this plant-based diet idea of yours and that's why I've come to see you again this morning."

"Is your family going to support you?" asked Gail.

"My wife is, yes. I've not mentioned it to my daughter Ellie yet. Is that important?"

"It's not essential," said Gail, "but from experience, I can tell you that having the support of your partner or family does make a big difference.

"So what can I eat" asked Peter.

"Much more than you think," said Gail. "Most of my clients often discover a wonderful world full of taste, texture and variety that they never imagined existed. A plant-based diet focuses on foods derived from plant sources. These can include fruit, vegetables, grains, pulses, legumes, nuts and meat substitutes, such as soy products. You'll be consuming a wide variety of fruits, vegetables and pulses *and* you'll have excellent intakes of fibre and the vitamins and minerals that are present in fruit and vegetables. I'll give you some information and ideas now on good healthy things that you can eat for breakfast, lunch and dinner and I'll include some ideas for snacks. I have a small diet pamphlet that I can give you to take home with you that will get you started and give you something better than dried toast to look forward to!"

"My wife will be pleased!" Peter said.

"I think it's best to keep breakfast simple. You're at the beginning of your journey, so a simple transition is key. I would recommend that you go to the supermarket and buy some oats, a milk alternative such as rice milk, almond milk or soya milk, some dried raisins, some frozen blue berries or your favourite variety of dark berries, some flax seed and some chia seeds. Then you just pour your plant milk onto the oats, add a table spoon of flax seeds and then add the other ingredients as you wish. This gives you a simple go-to breakfast that you can make within minutes. Of course, there are lots of other healthy breakfast options including chickpea omelette, polenta with pears and cranberries, brown rice breakfast pudding and hundreds of others. I'll help you over the coming weeks and months, but like I said, this oat breakfast will get you started and on your way."

"I bought some Soya milk the other day so I'll pour that on my porridge," said Peter, "so what about lunch?" I'm going back to work soon and I'll be out and about in the van and I don't want to go hungry."

"You're going to be doing a little bit of advance preparation," Gail replied. "Just like for breakfast, there are lots of healthy meals you can make, but because the wider world has not quite caught on to all the fantastic benefits of a plant-based diet, you're gong to want to prepare in advance. In the pamphlet that I mentioned, there are some links to websites with lots of suggestions for packed lunches and home-made lunches. Some of my favourite packed lunches include orange sesame quinoa salad, chickpea salad sandwiches, and roasted veggie quinoa bowl.

"But we don't want to make this too complicated at the beginning. There's a list of a few essentials that will make everything easier for you. You should stock up on these and make sure you always have them at home. These include wholegrain pasta, rice, beans, tofu, lentils, unsalted nuts of all varieties, frozen berries, oats, plant-based milks, dark chocolate - the darker the better - chickpeas, agave syrup, baked beans, broccoli, greens, fruit and vegetables. The rule for vegetables is, the darker the colour, the better it is. So, for instance, red cabbage is better than green cabbage because it's darker. The darker colour indicates that there are more anti-oxidants present.

"Momentum is key. Start small. Just find something that's healthy, tasty and filling for breakfast and stick to that until you're ready to start experimenting. The same applies for lunch, dinner and snacks. You're lucky because your timing is very good. The supermarkets have more choice and more plant-based options than ever before and the UK as got to be one of the best places in the world when it comes to plant-based choices and variety in the shops."

"Like anything else you want to learn for the first time, the most important thing is to work on the foundations and just get started. Concentrate on momentum and moving in the right direction. Even *I'm* learning new things everyday and that's fantastic. I promise you that if you stick with this you'll discover much more variety, taste and fun with your food than you can possible imagine now. Not only that, you can look forward to some other huge changes which at the moment you can't perceive but which you will experience like everyone else that switches to a plant-based diet."

"I feel ready," Peter said. "I hope I can do this."

"And remember," Gail said, "in nature, nothing is hurried, yet everything is achieved".

Feeling more positive and motivated, Peter thanked Gail for her advice and drove home. As soon as Susan returned from work, he wanted to go shopping for these new ingredients, most of which he'd never heard of before. *What the bloody hell are flax seeds?* he thought to himself.

Shopping this time with Susan was a slightly weird experience. For years they had routinely gone to the same supermarket for the weekly shopping and knew more or less exactly what they would be buying. The shopping for the entire week was often completed by the two of them in less than half an hour.

Today was different. It was strange to walk past all the produce and foods that they knew so well. In fact, apart from baked beans and one or two other things, the things that he and Susan were putting in their trolley today were completely new and novel, at least as far as they were concerned. And something else was happening, too. For the first time in his life, he started to notice what other people were putting in their trollies. Never in the past had the contents of other people's supermarket trollies interested him in the slightest. Today, however, after the events of the past couple of weeks and all the knowledge that had been revealed to him, he was noticing. He watched how others choose foods and products, which he now knew were harmful to health, animals and the environment, and became aware that many were being driven primarily by taste, price and convenience rather than what might be healthy or good for the planet. And just a few weeks ago, he had been exactly the same.

Peter thought again about his own Dad; he'd been diagnosed with heart disease when he was only 64 years old. He remembered how his dad, only a few years earlier before, had played football with Peter and a few mates. His Dad had managed to keep up with them on the pitch despite being 20 odd years older. That was before he retired. His Dad had been a plumber all his life and had been active. But after his retirement - which he'd looked forward to for so long - he became far less active. Especially in the dark winter months, his Dad had occupied himself watching TV. After four years of a predominately sedentary lifestyle, he'd started getting chest pains. He was diagnosed with heart disease. First he'd had a couple of stents fitted into his blocked arteries. The benefits of the stents had lasted only a couple of years before he started getting angina again. At age 67, Peter's father had had a triple heart bypass. The operation was long, but his stay in hospital wasn't. Peter thought back to the day when he'd gone to the hospital with his mother to collect his dad and bring him home.

Peter laughed to himself as he thought about his Dad's response to the leaflet that the hospital had given him on the day he went home. Peter cast his mind back to the very late afternoon on which his father had been discharged from hospital. Peter's mother was cooking an evening meal and Peter was in the living room talking to his father. Peter remembered leafing through the information from the hospital and saying to his dad, "It looks like you're going to have to change your diet, Dad"

"No, I don't," Peter's father had replied. "Everything it says in that leaflet I already do"

"No, you don't," Peter had said, "there is a chart in here that says at least a third of your diet should be fruit or vegetables"

"Apart from that," said Peter's Dad in all seriousness, "I do everything that it says in there."

Peter's father's bypass operation had saved his life. It really was miraculous. In the days before having the operation, he'd been short of breath, had pains in his chest, and was very unwell. The operation changed all that and improved his father's condition enormously. But Peter remembered the days, weeks and months after the operation, when the effects of the strong pain killers wore off. Peter's dad had suffered. The urgent threat to his life from heart disease had eased, but he bore out a whole year of pain and discomfort. Peter was determined that his own fate would be different than the one endured by his father.

"You've got nuts written down here," said Susan, looking down at the list Gail had given Peter. "Shall we go and get some of those first?"

Susan was becoming more and more impressed with her husband's determination each day. When she'd first told Peter about Michael running marathons, she'd done it without thinking. She'd certainly not expected the meeting to lead to anything. But she liked and was pleased by her husband's new-found direction. He'd told Susan about his plans to get fit enough to go out with his mates on a Sunday morning. She was still unsure whether he would follow through on his plans, but for now she was hopeful.

Standing in the queue for the supermarket checkout, Peter said, "It's like going shopping for the first time again, isn't it? Most of the things in our trolley we've never bought before." Susan laughed adding "and we've still not found out what flax seeds are".

The next day, Peter got up early. He'd been contemplating Gail's words about nature and taking it slowly. In the past, whenever he'd set himself a goal, his natural tendency had always been to throw himself into it wholeheartedly. He'd decided to start jogging a few times in the past, but his attempts had always ended in the same predictable way. He'd typically put on his running shoes, go out of the door and start running. He'd quickly be out of breath, pushing himself to continue until he couldn't run any longer. Maybe he'd keep this up for a few days or even a couple of weeks, but at some point he would just give up because he was simply getting no enjoyment out of it at all. This idea of Gail's that he should look at things with a longer perspective and take his time was a concept that he now found very appealing.

Peter made his breakfast and put on his walking shoes – some day in the future, they be his running shoes again. His objective was to walk from his house to the nearby children's playground at the top of a small hill, around 10 minutes away. He would walk to the park at whatever pace was comfortable, take a rest when he arrived, and walk back slowly to his house. This week, that was all that was needed; next week, he could add a little more distance and try to increase his speed. With his mobile phone that was strapped to his arm, he could track his pace, distance and heart rate.

Just the act of walking to the park gave him a sense of empowerment. Regardless of what happened now, he felt in control again and that was all he needed.

CHAPTER 9 : THE YOGI

Susan had been doing yoga for over two years. She'd started out of interest and because she'd heard that it would help her to get strong and flexible. She'd just turned up one Friday and asked to take part. Apart from the instructor, Dietmar, two years ago when she'd started there had only been 4 or 5 others there, all in their 40s and 50s. Although she'd not really known what to expect, Susan had been surprised by the slow pace of the lesson. They had started by sitting cross legged on the floor. Dietmar had told her to get as comfortable as she could and that they were going to practice meditation. He'd told the class to concentrate on their breath just behind the nose. Should they become aware of their mind thinking thoughts, they should return to concentrating on their breath. After 10 minutes they then started some breathing exercises, which left Susan feeling calm and energized. In the end, it took 30 minutes or so before the stretching exercises to begin, though Susan had been expecting them right from the start. The lesson ended with a balance exercise and the chanting of Aum (Om).

Several things, however, had surprised Susan about the lesson. It had been a peaceful yet energizing experience. She'd realized that her body was not as flexible as she thought, certainly not in comparison to the others in the class. But it was more than that; there had been something spiritual about the experience that she'd enjoyed. The slow pace, the silence and the awareness of her body. The 90-minute yoga session had been like a retreat from the rest of the world. She liked it. Going to yoga on Monday and Friday evening was now a part of her regular routine. She'd also integrated a short session of meditation and yoga into her morning routine and had discovered that getting up early and completing a short routine before the rest of the world woke up, left her feeling in control and ready for the day to begin.

Susan thought that yoga would also benefit Peter. She'd noticed the groaning sounds that he now made when bending over and knew that he was losing his flexibility. She'd decided to ask him again when the right moment presented itself.

The door opened and Peter walked in having successfully walked to the park and back.

"That went well," he said.

"Did you get any chest pains? Was your breathing OK?" asked Susan.

"All good," said Peter. "I should have started this years ago"

Peter bent over to untie his shoelaces and let out a groan.

"You're making noises like an old man!" said Susan. "Are you sure you don't want to come with me to Yoga? It would fix all those OAP noises that you're making."

It had not slipped Peter's attention that his wife Susan had really taken to doing yoga. He was intrigued by her new-found discipline. She'd get out of bed early to sit meditating before practicing some yoga stretches. On the one hand, he thought that it might be good for the two of them to do something together twice a week. But on the other hand, Peter believed Yoga to be a women's thing and definitely not something in which a man of his generation would willingly participate. Sure, he'd noticed that his body was stiffening up and he'd had a nagging pain in the small of his back for years. The doctor had told him there was nothing wrong and that it was just part of aging. *But I'm only 53 years old*, he thought to himself. Years ago Susan had persuaded Peter to go to dance classes. During the course of around three years they'd learned a wide variety of dances including cha-cha-cha, rumba, waltz, Viennese walz, jive, tango and samba. He'd gone more for Susan than himself and although the dance lessons had been alright once he was there, he'd never looked forward to going and was glad when they stopped. Whenever Susan mentioned going to yoga, he equated it with ballroom dancing.

"Michael thought that it would help his running and it doesn't seem to have done his recovery any harm. Maybe it would help you in the same way," said Susan.

Peter pictured Michael in his mind. He'd only met him the one time, but he certainly made a positive impact on him. Michael the Marathon Runner was calm, focused and clearly determined. "Oh, alright then", said Peter, "I'll come on Friday and give it a try, but I'm not promising anything. It's just a test."

"You're going to Yoga, Dad?" Ellie laughed. "Will you be able to do a headstand soon?"

"I'm only going to one session to see what it's like, that's all. Anyway, what did your teacher say about the meeting that we had the other night?" Peter was keen to change the subject.

"She said that it's very difficult to get people to change their habits," said Ellie. "She said something about culture and tradition being incredibly powerful forces and told me to concentrate on things that people might actually do."

Peter said, "that's a bit pessimistic. I mean, you're the next generation, so I think the school should be at least telling you about it. Whether you do anything about it is a different thing, but at least you would have the knowledge."

"Forget it, Dad," said Ellie.

The following Friday Peter went with Susan to his first yoga class. They arrived a little early and were just getting out of the car when Michael spoke from behind them. "Hello", he said. "Both of you today".

"I'm just going to give it a go for now to see if I like it", said Peter.

"It would be nice to have another man join us. There's only Dietmar and me among all the women."

"Dietmar's our age, too, isn't he?", said Peter.

"He's in his 50s. He's been doing yoga for donkey's years and has been to India a few times to improve and learn more.", said Michael. He's a big believer in the spiritual side of yoga, which in actual fact is what yoga is all about."

"But it costs him students", said Susan. "Most people come to do stretching and when they find out it's actually about meditation through breathing and stretching, they lose interest".

Peter arrived at the yoga hall feeling like a fish out of water. Everything in the hall was made from wood including the natural untreated wooden floor. In the corner there was a basket containing the yoga mats and a faint smell of incense filled the air.

Dietmar walked over to Peter and shook his hand.

"Nice to see you here this evening," he said, "I hope you enjoy it. Susan's told me about your health scare and that you're on a mission to try and get better without surgery. I think that yoga might help you, too, just like it did Michael."

"I'm here more out of curiosity than anything. I don't think yoga can help my heart," said Peter.

"You're mistaken", said Dietmar, confidently. "I bet you didn't know that there are academic studies about the ways that yoga may help heart disease risk as much as going for a brisk walk."

Yoga's unique because it combines physical activity, breathing, and meditation. Each of these positively affects your heart, so combining them is bound to be beneficial. When we practice the yoga postures, your muscles are gently stretched and exercised, making them more sensitive to insulin, which is important for blood sugar levels. We also do deep breathing which lowers blood pressure and our mind-calming meditation quiets the nervous system and eases stress. And don't forget that practicing yoga seriously means adopting a vegetarian or vegan diet, which have also been proven to help with heart disease. Eating meat is bad Karma."

"So I've been hearing," Peter joked.

"When you meet people that have cut out all animal products from their diet and ask them whether they've noticed any changes, what do you think is the most common reply by far?"

"They slim down?" said Peter.

"A sense of calm," Dietmar replied. "It that makes a lot of sense if you think about it. When you eat meat, you also eat the bad energy and violence that went into creating it. Just think how we treat animals. At the point of slaughter animals are terrified and anxious and this energy is transferred into their bodies, which we later eat. Is it really any wonder that anxiety rates in the West are going through the roof? I wish people would think more about the actions that they take. I was watching a program on TV the other night about cruelty-free farming. There was an expert on animal behaviour on the panel and he believes that our entire society is plagued with this low-level guilty conscience about eating meat. This leads us all to be more violent and anxious than we are by nature. This is the price that we pay for eating animals. But you're here now for the first time, so you're obviously opening your mind to new things."

"I don't know if Susan's already told you, but we're switching to a plant-based diet, so that part is not going to be difficult," said Peter. "I've certainly been opening my mind to new realities over the past few weeks, more by necessity than choice. To be fair, I'm only here to try it out, so don't expect me to become a regular".

"You say that," said Dietmar, "but how many other people in your situation would have just chosen the usual path and carried on as normal? You're standing here now in front of me about to take your first yoga class. That means something. Anyway, let's get started. Take your time and just do what you can do. The most important thing for your first class is to feel comfortable and try to get used to being here. Try to soak up a bit of the environment and energy and imagine how far you might be able to go."

Peter walked over to the basket, picked out a mat and laid it on the floor. The others were also using a folded blanket to sit on to add height while sitting cross legged, so he got one too. Peter thought to himself that he hadn't sat crossed legged on the floor since he was about 9 years old for school assembly. That was over 40 years ago. As he crossed his legs he instantly felt uncomfortable, but decided to ignore it for now. The class took 90 minutes, yet to Peter the time seemed to pass fairly quickly, albeit at slow pace. His body felt good after all this stretching. His mind also seemed clearer, but he still wasn't sure whether he wanted to continue.

"Well," said Susan, "What did you think? Want to come again on Monday?"

"We'll see," said Peter.

CHAPTER 10 : THE TURNING POINT

Two months after Peter's diagnosis, he was on a strict plant-based diet and exercising every day. He felt better. And there was something else, something that he'd first noticed in the supermarket. Peter had start to see and think about the world differently! He'd started to question how he could have been so blind and ignorant for so long. He thought of himself as being fairly intelligent, but he'd completely missed the blatantly obvious injustice and cruelty carried out on animals every day. Talk about elephant in the room - this was more like a mammoth! Now he could see it. On every street corner there were posters promoting meaty fast-food, huge signs with images of burgers. Meat and animal products were promoted everywhere. There was so much of it that it was hardly surprising that people didn't even think twice. And neither had he.

In effect, he'd now adopted a vegan lifestyle in an effort to return to health. He'd always thought of vegans as being extreme hippies and weird. But he was now also vegan, and he was realizing more every day that it was, in fact, wider society and everyone else that was extreme. He now thought that participating in the mistreatment and slaughter of animals for no other reason than to enjoy a fleeting nice taste in your mouth was extreme and weird. And it was everywhere. Peter now understood that he could never turn back, regardless of how his heart-disease problem ended.

By eating only plant-based foods, Peter had given up on many of the foods that he had known all his life. But in return he had won so much more. He was discovering this huge world of other things that he could eat that also tasted delicious. He was now actively improving his health and his chances of living longer; he was no longer part of the proxy violence that was taking place every day on animals and he was making a significant contribution to preventing the destruction of the planet. And there was more: Dietmar was right. Peter had also noticed that he felt calmer than he had before.

After six months had passed since Peter's diagnosis, his morning walk had expanded slowly day by day; he was even at a point where he could break into a very gentle run. Peter was no longer getting short of breath, had no chest pains, and felt better than he had in years. His diet had changed completely and he'd become quite obsessed with making sure he was getting all the nutrition and variety that Gail had recommended. Not only that, but he was doing yoga twice a week!

Men are simple creatures and so it was that Peter took the most delight from the fact that he'd started noticing his penis coming back to life. He'd almost forgot the delightful sensations of getting an erection or semi-erection in everyday situations. It had been months since Peter had enjoyed a good session in bed with Susan and he was beginning to feel up to it in more ways than one. *Let's see if we can make it happen this weekend*, he thought to himself.

Peter had e-mailed his cardiologist months ago telling him that he'd decided against surgery. He'd explained that he was going to try an alternative plant-based approach. Peter was feeling so much better that he wanted to join the lads on Sunday mornings for a hike in the Peak District. That's what Peter had been working his way towards and was really looking forward to it.

It was time to go back to the cardiologist and get a check up.

Dr. Newton had been looking forward to seeing Peter again. He'd been surprised by Peter's message in which he asked to cancel the bypass operation. None of his patients had ever taken such a decision before when faced with the alternative. It had been over six months since he'd last seen Peter and he was taken aback by his appearance as he walked into the office.

"Well, you're certainly looking better than the last time we met," said Dr. Newton.

"Thank you. I'm feeling better in every way," said Peter.

After a few tests, Dr. Newton sat Peter down to talk.

"Well," he said, "the blockages in your veins have eased, your cholesterol levels have dropped significantly and you've clearly lost a lot of weight. You tell me that you're feeling better and - given today's findings - I can understand why. Can you explain to me what you've been doing and how you've managed to ease your heart disease without my help?"

Peter was glad to share as much as he could about the events of the past six months with Dr. Newton, and the advice that he'd been given by Gail the nutritionist.

Dr. Newton had been practicing cardiology for the past twenty eight years; in all that time, he'd never witnessed anything like this. Of course, as a cardiologist he was acutely aware that diet and lifestyle play a huge role in *causing* heart disease and personally he believed that up to 80% of his patients at least had conditions linked to lifestyle and diet. Until now, however, he'd never considered that diet and lifestyle could also play a role in *curing* it. Controlling it, maybe, but curing it?? This was something new.

Peter could see that Dr. Newton was a little lost for words.

"My Nutritionist is called Gail and she told me that medical students complain that they learn almost nothing about the way diet and lifestyle affect health", said Peter. "She also told me that even doctors that are aware of the data are reluctant to tell their patients because they don't think that they would be prepared to make the changes necessary. To be fair, if I think about my dad, who also had heart disease, that's true. There's no way that he would have made the changes. But, as you can see, there are some people who are ready to try a different approach because they want to bypass the bypass surgery. "

Peter couldn't wait to get home to tell Susan and Ellie the good news, but first he decided to go to see Gail and tell her what his results had shown. Walking into her office, he could see that she was taken by surprise.

"I don't want to take up much of your time," said Peter to Gail. "I've just come by to say thank you. Without your advice and faith in your method, I would probably be sitting at home now with my veins and blood full of pain killers, statins and whatever the else the hospital would have given me after my surgery. But instead, I'm going to meet up with my mates on Sunday morning and we're going for a hike in the Peak District. How brilliant is that? I've lost weight, but more than that - I feel far more compassionate, calm and in harmony with the world. And it's been far easier than I thought, but maybe I've been lucky because Susan has been very supportive and helped me follow though on the changes. She's even managed to persuade me to go to yoga with her twice a week. The next time someone comes to you that is unsure and you have the feeling that he or she just needs living proof that your approach can work, just send them over to me and I'll tell them and show them what's possible."

Gail smiled as she replied, "Thank you for your kind words. They motivate me even more! I hope you persist and reap even more benefits over the years."

That Friday night, Peter treated Susan by reserving a table in their favourite vegan restaurant. One of the surprising things he'd discovered about eating plants is that no two dishes are ever the same. When he'd first contemplated eating a purely plant-based diet, he expected to lose a lot of choice and variety. In fact, the opposite had occurred. He was now eating and enjoying foods that he'd never realized existed before. The food in this particular restaurant was simply delicious. He'd booked his table early, knowing just how busy they get – he never would have imagined a place like this being full before!

"Who would have thought a year ago that we'd be sitting in a place like this?" said Susan, after they'd ordered their meal.

"I know," said Peter. "It's almost like we've done a complete reset and started again. Dr. Newton told me that I've improved significantly and that he'd never seen such progress before. I just had to see Gail and thank her."

The waitress came over and poured them both a glass of red wine and set down some water.

"I also want thank you, Susan," he continued. "I'm not sure I would have been able to have seen though all these changes without you making them, too. I hope it's not been too much of a sacrifice for you."

"Not at all," said Susan. "It's one of the best things that's happened to me and perhaps to us for a long time. I felt as though we were drifting apart. Before you used to get back from work and have very little interest in anything, including me. I'd ask you to join me for yoga, but you weren't interested. I didn't enjoy seeing you sitting there watching TV and not doing a lot else apart from work. I still can't believe how much you've changed in such a short time."

"Neither can I," said Peter reaching across the table to take Susan's hand.

It was a lovely evening for them both. The wine helped, it was true, but it had been years since they'd talked so openly with each other. Arriving home, they both took off their shoes and kissed. Peter felt a reassuring arousal.

I'm back, he said to himself with an inward grin.

Susan had noticed, too.

"It feels like you're back in action," she said, laughing as they pressed their bodies close. "Shall we see what you've got?"

"Good idea," Peter replied, kissing her as they disappeared into the bedroom.

Peter was a new man and a real man.

The End.

ABOUT THE AUTHOR

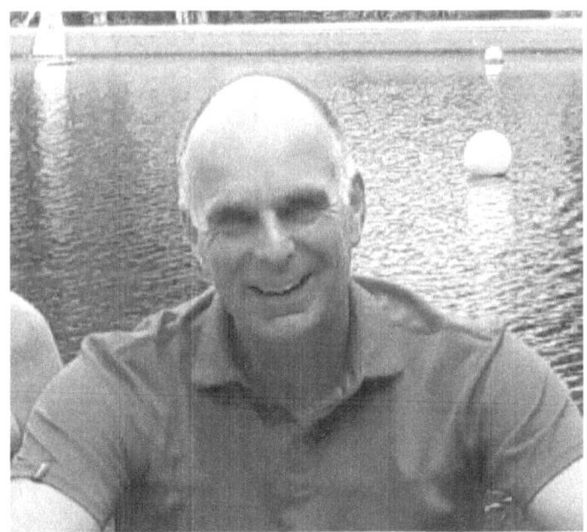

Alan Twigg speaks English, German and Spanish and is the International Author of "And Suddenly, Everything Changed", which is published in print and audio in English and German.

Born and raised in Sheffield in the north of England, Alan spent 18 years in Germany and now lives in Tenerife in the Canary Islands. A successful Entrepreneur, his professional life has been rich and varied from working in a gas station to international haulage and from translating to being the Managing Director and Owner of an Internet Marketing Agency near Stuttgart, Germany.

A father of four children and already a grandfather, he's also a passionate golfer, dancer of Argentine tango and practitioner of meditation and yoga.

Acknowledgement

Thank you to my wonderful daughter Lea for nudging and nudging me into the world of plant-based eating for the sake of the sentient animals, my health and the planet. Thank you love.

Disclaimer

This is a work of fiction. Names, characters, businesses, places, events, locales, and incidents are either the products of the author's imagination or used in a fictitious manner. Any resemblance to actual persons, living or dead, or actual events is purely coincidental.

This book is not intended as a substitute for the medical advice of physicians. The reader should regularly consult a physician in matters relating to his/her health and particularly with respect to any symptoms that may require diagnosis or medical attention.

I hope you enjoyed "And Suddenly, Everything Changed". Please write a review so others can find this book more easily.

www.ingramcontent.com/pod-product-compliance
Lightning Source LLC
Chambersburg PA
CBHW051216250726
48655CB00006B/2439